Living with Pick's

A Diary of Life-Changing Events

Ian Faraday

Copyright © Ian Faraday 2024

All rights reserved. No part of this book may be reproduced or transmitted in any form or by any means without written permission from the author.

Table of Contents

Acknowledgements i
About the Author iii
The Next Stages 5
After That 9
Ever On! 12
The Next Instalment 15
Here We Go Again 19
One More Step 22
More and More 26
Extracts From a Newsletter To Friends and Family 31
Up to Date 48
2014 57
2015 60
2015 63
2016 67
2017 71
2018 74
2019 76
2020 78
2021 81
2022 84
2023 86

2024.. 89
In Conclusion - 2024.. 93

Dedication

This book is dedicated to Little El - my beautiful late wife Elspeth - and all those who may be affected in any way by a similar illness.

Acknowledgements

Grateful thanks to Ruairidh Greig, Ruth Midgley, Wendy Haggett, and my cousins David and Mary Shaw for their valuable assistance in proofreading the script. Also to my daughter Alice for the cover photograph and my good friend PJ for his very useful recommendations.

About the Author

Ian Faraday was born in Morecambe, England, and moved to Sheffield in 1969 to train as a teacher, specialising in French and Music. He has written a variety of songs for children and young people, many of which have been published.

His interest in writing stories for children began with a time-travelling adventure entitled 'The Magic Path' and this was followed by three sequels in the same series.

Some years ago, Ian's wife Elspeth was diagnosed with a form of early-onset dementia known as Pick's Disease. This gave him the opportunity to write a very different book, which tells the story of how the illness progressed and how the family and many different agencies dealt with Elspeth's slow deterioration from start to finish.

Ian has two daughters and two grandchildren. His main interests, other than writing, are playing the piano and working with a local Youth Theatre.

It was April 2012 when I began writing this account, and my wife Elspeth was fifty-nine years old. She had been diagnosed with 'frontotemporal lobar degeneration' (FTD) or 'Pick's Disease' about five years before this date. I want to tell this story so that anyone who may be interested can learn about this rare disease, for which, sadly, there is no known cure.

Back at that time, and probably to this day, not many people had heard of Pick's Disease. It is a severe form of early-onset dementia, which generally hits younger people between the ages of about forty to sixty. There will, of course, be exceptions to this. It is caused by a build-up of protein in the brain.

Elspeth Mirren Cramond Greig and I were married in 1976 on our shared birthday, August the 5th, though I was three years older. I was born in Morecambe in 1949, and she in Cleethorpes in 1952. I still have my wedding suit, with speech and confetti in the pockets! What a pity it no longer fits, though it might be a little out of fashion now! Elspeth was a jewellery designer who trained at the Art College in Sheffield, and I was a teacher. She was an incredibly practical person and had many skills, ranging from sewing to bricklaying or painting (of all kinds), cooking, gardening, and virtually anything. We have two amazing daughters, Catriona and Alice, who I still call 'my girls', even though today, in 2024, they are forty-one and thirty-nine years old!

Elspeth was always a good conversationalist and storyteller, particularly at the dinner table. In about 2002, when speaking, she started to 'ramble on', and it was clear that friends were putting up with her because they knew and liked her. Her behaviour started to alter.

She began to go on long walks and bus trips; sometimes, these lasted the whole day. She took hundreds of photos and bought postcards wherever she went – all very tasteful, it must be said. There are at least a dozen albums of her pictures here at home today and around fifteen hundred postcards, which she collected on her travels!

She began to pick up other things. She brought vast quantities of empty milk bottles home from her walks in the countryside, washing them meticulously and storing them all over the house. Once, I took two batches of about a hundred and twenty bottles back to a local dairy. Staff there were more than a little surprised when I told them my wife had 'found' some milk bottles. I kept on bringing bag after bag of them in from the car! About the same number were back at home, washed and stored neatly in cupboards. She also collected lollipop sticks, plastic cocktail stirrers, sweet wrappers, notebooks, red and green plastic clothes pegs for Christmas cards and many other small and trivial items. She began to turn lights off randomly at home; she drew the curtains and blinds in the middle of the day; she closed car windows and house windows, even on the hottest of days, when others wanted them open; she would march straight to the front of the queue at supermarkets and tell people not to buy cigarettes as they shouldn't be smoking - I had to ring the manager to apologise on a number of occasions; she turned taps on in the bathroom and left them running, causing water to pour through the floor and into the kitchen below; she began turning the gas oven on and walking away without it being lit, also turning the oven off when something was cooking! We had to guess how much time remained for the meal to be properly cooked! Family and friends mistakenly thought her actions might be due to the menopause. We really felt it was time to go to our GP when a couple of very strange things happened.

Elspeth took to walking into Sheffield city centre, following the railway track which ran near our house. One day, a train driver saw her doing this, and he thought she was too close to the track, thereby putting herself in danger. He reported her to the railway police, who stopped her and 'arrested' her. She did not understand what was happening, so she struggled. The officers, who knew nothing of her condition (and neither did anyone else yet), brought her home in plastic handcuffs. She could not work out why they had done this. My younger daughter Alice was at home when the police arrived with Elspeth. I was out but came home after Alice rang me to tell me what had happened. I spoke with the police and explained the situation, which prompted an apology for the handcuffs.

The other event which alarmed us was that she found a vodka half-bottle in the countryside and told us that she had drunk the remaining few drops, oblivious to the possible consequences. Shortly after this incident, I took her to our GP, who did some tests and sent her to the hospital for scans. The MRI scan showed some brain deterioration. The Consultant gave us information about Pick's Disease and a leaflet about Power of Attorney, but I didn't really understand much of what she said. Elspeth didn't care. She went off into Sheffield with a wet patch on the back of her skirt, saying it would dry by itself. She refused the offered urine test.

Elspeth was still doing some cooking at this time, but there were signs that her ability in this field was declining. Usually, just like her mother, she cooked a fabulous Christmas dinner, but one year, nothing worked. The turkey was not cooked, and the stuffing was like sawdust, similar to the pudding. She started to lose interest in all the things she enjoyed. She began to go to bed early and sleep for twelve hours, which was something she had never done before. She stopped doing household jobs and left everything to me. I think it was in about 2008 that the Community Psychiatric Nurse (CPN) began to visit us to offer advice. The Alzheimer's Society and two other care agencies became involved and looked after Elspeth while I was at school. I was a junior school Deputy Head, but I gave that up and went down to three, then two days a week, retiring early, partly to help look after her and partly to continue (from home) my new career of working for a school's music firm based in Market Harborough. I am still involved with them today, writing and scoring musicals for the primary age range. I have so much to thank the director for since he gave me the opportunity to work for his company. Over the years, this has given me a valuable break from thinking too much about the difficulties at home.

So that's how Elspeth's illness began. I hope I have started to give you some sort of insight into what was becoming such a challenging situation. After twenty-five years our life together was changing rapidly. I made up my mind that I would just have to get used to it and do my best, although I had no idea what was to come.

The Next Stages

(First written late April 2012)

The Alzheimer's Society sent staff to our house on three mornings in the week. At this point I was still able to leave Elspeth for a few minutes, doing a jigsaw puzzle while I went to school. The Outreach carers arrived and let themselves in, using a key which was 'hidden' in a key safe next to the garage. However, it was not long before we decided, for safety reasons, that Elspeth could not be left on her own, and two care agencies entered the scene. Because of the seriousness of her illness, we were granted funding for quite a few hours a week, on average about eight hours per day. I took over for the other sixteen, which included the night shift. Carers took Elspeth out whenever possible, as she still very much enjoyed going for a drive or a walk.

Soon, she began to do even stranger things, which were sometimes dangerous. When out in the car, she would open the door while it was moving and sometimes try to get out. She would pull up the handbrake and play with the steering wheel and indicators while the car was being driven. She was soon banished to the back seats, and child locks were put on.

Because Elspeth had enjoyed bus trips in the past, one carer tried to continue with this activity. Outings had to stop when Elspeth began shutting windows and being extra noisy. Equally enigmatic was her behaviour at home. She turned the television off when people were watching it. I also remember, one night, when senior managers from one care agency came to discuss her care package, she turned all the lights off in the front room, went out and shut the door, leaving us all in the dark! On another occasion, one afternoon, I was cleaning our bedroom window while standing on a small extension outside. She came into the bedroom, looked at me and immediately shut and locked the window! She then left the room without a word. Fortunately, our carer heard me banging on the window and came upstairs to rescue me and let me back in.

Elspeth began to eat everything in sight. Firstly, a dozen apples or carrots in a day, and a similar number of bananas, then lots of bread and chocolate. She drank many cups of coffee, one after the other. She took food out of the fridge, eating any large pots of yoghurt. Oddly, she went into the waste bin and put waste food back into the fridge, which, if not spotted, could have proved dangerous. It was not long before we locked the food away in the garage and properly regulated her diet.

Despite the walking she was doing, Elspeth put on a lot of weight, though this might have been partly due to the anti-psychotic tablets which she was taking daily.

She next went through a period of recording hundreds of gas and electric meter readings, filling many notebooks from her vast collection. All the figures were written in neat columns, with date and time. She kept a daily diary, which she wrote when she went to bed, telling of her excursions. It tended to always say the same sort of things, and each sentence ended with the word 'yes!' followed by an exclamation mark. All these books are still in our bedside drawer.

Elspeth did not seem to recognise anyone, even lifelong friends from her childhood. Her mother, Sheila, had always been her best friend, but all Elspeth could say on our visits to the care home in Grimsby where Mother was staying was, *'Is that my mother?'* before proceeding to walk along the corridors, turning off all the lights in the rooms, much to the occupant's annoyance. On the plus side, she was closely followed by my daughter Catriona, who was switching them all back on again and apologising to the complaining ladies! We went home early that day. Granny died not long after this. When I told Elspeth her mother had passed away, she just said, *'Did they bury her in the ground?'* And that was it. She showed no understanding of what had happened and took no interest in the funeral.

I must just mention again that before her illness, Elspeth was a trained jewellery designer and maker. She made beautiful gold, silver and platinum items, including our wedding rings, one in 9 and the other in 18-carat gold. She had her own hallmark, so the rings were hallmarked at the Sheffield Assay Office. In 1976, the rings, together, cost us less than £20! I can't fit mine onto my finger any more, but my daughter Alice keeps her mother's engagement and wedding rings safe and enjoys wearing them on special occasions. The engagement ring is rather lovely. We bought this on Steep Hill in Lincoln for £100. Elspeth was never a fan of diamonds, so she chose one with three opals, which flashed colour when at different angles.

Before her illness, Elspeth spent five years working for a jewellery firm in Sheffield. When our children came along, she left the firm and worked from home, making items for craft fairs, such as cheaper jewellery and lots of hand-painted wooden badges, the latter being mainly named teddy bears in various outfits. She actually made over a hundred of these for the nurses at Sheffield Children's Hospital. She also did calligraphy work on medical certificates for Sheffield University. One day, she found that she could not control her hands as well as usual. She had pains in the base of her neck and arms. After tests, she was diagnosed with two extra ribs at the top of her spine. Although she learnt to live with this, it was clear that it really bothered her. The alternative was a dicey operation to remove the ribs. I often wonder, maybe fancifully, whether the pressure on the base of her neck contributed some way to her illness. Those who are medically knowledgeable may disagree with this, but it is just an idea I had. She never made or painted anything else since that time.

After That

(First written April 2012)

I'm going to deal with the delicate matter of continence now. It's actually connected with jigsaw puzzles, if you can believe that!

Elspeth began squatting to urinate on her walks. It did not seem to matter where she was or who was watching. People out strolling in public parks would have been quite shocked. They, of course, did not know her. Carers did their best with this situation but soon, the walk venues had to be changed to less populated areas. At home, she started to go to the toilet many times a day, often with no results. The noise of the toilet flushing became a regular sound at our home. You can guess that the house water bill more than doubled! We even tried to lock the doors and regulate her visits, but she then urinated in the bath, carefully swilling everything away with the shower attachment. We gave that idea up quickly!

We next took her for a urine test to see if there was an infection. This could have been quite difficult, but she had taken to using a plastic jug in the pantry when she did not want to reach the toilet. We rescued the jug one day and took the sample to the surgery—negative result. The doctor asked for a second sample. The negative result again. Now, the connection with jigsaws follows.

The winter of 2010/11 was very snowy in Sheffield. My car was under a couple of feet of snow in the driveway. That was bad for our carers, as they had great difficulty getting to our house (we lived halfway up a long, steep hill), but they always made it, often leaving their cars at the bottom. The worry was whether we could think of activities for Elspeth if she was not able to go out for a drive or a walk. She did not see any dangers with walking in the snow, so she continuously asked to go out. We knew she enjoyed doing crosswords. Her novel way of completing them was to look up answers and write them in! In time, this changed to putting in meaningless words – ones that actually looked like words but were not, such as *'theephelcphpelad'* or *'enjolthen'*. She was tired of this activity in about half an hour. Then we discovered jigsaws. She very much enjoyed doing them, in particular the ones for seven to eight-year-olds, with a hundred extra-large pieces. A bit different from when I remember her doing jigsaws of one thousand or more tiny pieces with ease. She would sit for hours, absorbed. Everyone became quite interested in 'jigsawing' with her (it's addictive), but she was the best at it. A new jigsaw would take her a while to put together, but the ones she was used to did not take very long at all. She never needed the pattern on the box. I enjoyed looking on the internet for different jigsaws and bought a new one every now and then. For a year or so, she loved doing these puzzles until she began to last for about ten seconds before wanting to stand up and walk about. I remember every time she finished one, she would stand up and say, *'Am I going to the toilet now?'* Every time! Nothing would get in her way. She was very strong, which caused problems for smaller carers. I used to tell her she had only just been to the loo, but she was determined to go and often pushed me off balance – not maliciously, of course. So, the jigsaws and continence problems were closely connected!

Unfortunately, around this time, things deteriorated further, and she started to be brought home from walks very wet. She gave up the idea of squatting, obviously finding it easier to urinate in her clothes and soiling her underwear. She had to come home and be changed before being taken out again. We had a visit from the Sheffield Continence Team, who sorted her out with appropriate protection, providing her with monthly pad deliveries. I must point out that Elspeth was given several baths a week, which helped greatly with her personal hygiene. Bathing was a job reserved for carers or myself.

Readers may be wondering what effect all this was having on our family. Well, we saw it as having two choices. Either give up and become miserable because there is no cure for Pick's disease, and our mum may not be with us for many more years. Or we continue our lives in the best way possible and make sure we look after this talented and brilliant lady, giving her the very best care we could manage. In 1976, at our wedding, I made a promise to do the latter, and I was not going to break my word. The girls and I adopted a new family motto – 'Never Give Up' - ('Non Deficere' for Latin scholars!). The choice was not difficult.

Ever On!

(First written May 2012)

This was the most challenging part of my life. It was also the most frustrating. When Elspeth was 'granted' an enhanced care package, I believed that due to the gravity of her illness, she would have funded care for the rest of her life. If the details of this devastating illness were correct, that might be between two and twelve years, though opinions and websites somewhat differ. Most of her care came from myself and our two daughters, Catriona and Alice. Having carers call daily enabled me to look after Elspeth at home after they had finished, with somewhat more energy than if we were doing the full twenty-four-hour stint. I have much sympathy, and feel greatly for those families in a similar situation to us. Funded care is a tricky subject, and I understand that money has to be found from somewhere, but there are so many deserving cases.

For some years our cover was funded by Continuing Healthcare (CHC). To me, that seemed entirely right after paying a lifetime of taxes, etc. – and this was a rare and serious illness which could only worsen. The care package was reduced. There were months of uncertainty, arguing against this, and it reached the 'Appeals' stage. As part of this process, we had a meeting where Elspeth's current state was assessed, using a document called a 'Decision Support Tool' or 'DST' as it is known in the trade. The meeting was held here at home and attended by health visitors, care agency representatives, the NHS, and a member of the Sheffield Alzheimer's Society. The most important categories discussed, as far as Elspeth was concerned, were

Behaviour, Cognition, Communication and Continence. There were several others for which she would have lower or no needs. The big argument was over her behaviour – the top rating is severe. Two severe categories and the NHS would provide full funding. She was assessed as having severe behaviour at a previous meeting, but now the weighting was dropped to 'high'. This is a woman who would put herself into life-threatening situations. She needed twenty-four-hour care and could not be left alone.

Those connected with Elspeth's care would confirm that her behaviour could be extremely challenging and would often pose risks to Elspeth herself and, on occasion, to other people. Did a person have to show a violent temperament to exhibit severe behaviour? Elspeth was by no means violent, but her behaviour was severe in other ways. For example, she would walk up to strangers and adjust their clothing or even go off by herself and get into a stranger's car. She attempted to do these things a number of times, though, thankfully, the situation was dealt with by her carers.

Elspeth was unpredictable. We often did not know what she was going to do next. She had no real sense of danger – she would walk into the road if not stopped. Both she and passing motorists would clearly be in danger. Her carers had to be ready to cope with a variety of dangerous situations which might occur at any time. I once left the garage door open accidentally when she went to the garage toilet. I was distracted when the phone rang, and the next thing I knew, she had disappeared. After a frantic search, I found her striding down a nearby street in her slippers!

Further instances of her unpredictability occurred in the evening and during the night. She would put the bedroom light on at any hour, singing tunelessly and saying, *'Am I going downstairs?'* She would pick up her continence pants and tear them up, using her teeth. Sometimes, at any hour, she would get out of bed, get dressed and ask for breakfast or to go out for a drive. It started to be very wearing but it all needed dealing with.

As far as cognition was concerned, Elspeth had very severe needs. If there had been a higher level she would have been in it. She had short and long-term memory problems (she had no conversation and did not understand what other people said to her); she was often disorientated (she confused mealtimes with bedtimes, did not understand it was time to get washed/bathed/dressed, etc.); she could not make decisions or assess risks; we had to make sure her drinks were cool, as she often drank whatever we gave her straight down without a thought as to whether it was hot or cold. She became more and more reliant on the twenty-four-hour help she received from others. Looking at the Communication category on the DST at that time, apart from telling us she wanted to go to the toilet (when she often didn't want to go), she could not communicate her needs. She simply could not tell us what she wanted.

In the Continence category, the situation worsened considerably. As previously mentioned, Elspeth used to squat anywhere to urinate but that changed to just soiling herself without warning. We tried to anticipate this by asking her if she wanted to use the toilet, but that didn't work. The NHS Continence team visited us again and issued her with much bigger and more absorbent pads, which helped the situation until she started taking them off! We could not legislate for this and could not stop her from doing it. The arrival of continence pull-ups brought more success, but her nightdress was often soiled, likewise the bedclothes. The washing machine had to put in a lot of overtime!

The Next Instalment

(First written September 2012)

There was not a lot to report on the funding scene until the NHS Eligibility Panel met again. This group made decisions regarding funding and we were still waiting for the outcome. I wanted some definite information, but things seemed to drag on for months. Elspeth now had a care package of fifty-five hours weekly. It seemed ages before we were informed that the funding would be split between Health and Social Services. The NHS would fund one agency for twenty-two hours a week, and the cost of the other thirty-three hours would be split between Social Services and Elspeth. I had been e-mailing managers, who I hoped would deal with my concerns, as I needed to know how much we would be paying. Without the funding we had been receiving, the possible costs were very worrying if we wanted to keep the whole package. An NHS representative came to our house to discuss matters with me, and I was told that the NHS had been 'over-generous' with their original funding, so I knew we owed money, probably thousands, and I braced myself for a big bill landing on the doorstep before Christmas. We now had a very good Social Worker, who visited us and was trying to sort out a very complicated situation sooner rather than later. Nothing was definite yet. So, what of Elspeth? Her illness could only get worse, but due to an increase in her morning quetiapine tablet, she was a little calmer than before. Not always, but there had been a noticeable difference in her over the past weeks.

<u>This was a typical day:-</u>

Elspeth woke any time from 5.45 am onwards but generally later than that. When she woke, she would get up to go to the toilet and then want to go downstairs. She would look out of the bedroom window and say things such as, *'Ian's car is in the drive!'* Or, looking at the houses across the road, *'They called it a bungalow because they bunged a low roof on it!'* I had to get up with her and encourage her back to bed, where I would hang on to her arm until just before 7.00 am. At this time, she would often say, *'Am I going to the toilet?'* After this I would make sure she had washed her hands before she went downstairs. She would wander around, rattling the kitchen door every five minutes. There might be a period where she did a jigsaw, laid out on the dining room table the night before. She would not seem to recognise me when I gave her breakfast, but she accepted the food and always ate it, though sometimes it needed a lot of patience and encouragement on my part. At about 8.30 am, we went back upstairs to wash and dress. This took a lot of doing because she was now totally confused over what was happening. Toothbrush and flannel were laid out for her, but she often ignored them, asking whether she was going back to bed. Several reminders and a certain amount of help had to be given until success was achieved. She had to be helped to dress herself – she did not like taking her nightie off, which was not surprising, considering she was confronted by someone she probably did not know. When half-dressed, she would put her nightie or dressing gown back on and try to go back to bed. Changing Elspeth's continence pants was not the most pleasant task!

Next, we would go downstairs to finish breakfast and await the 9 o'clock carer. Getting her up was always something of an epic struggle. The carer arrived and probably did another jigsaw with Elspeth. As soon as a drive was mentioned, she would become very lively and vocal, often pushing her way past carers to reach the door. Doors would be locked otherwise she would be out and off, as had happened before. She would try to go barefoot or in her slippers on a rainy day. If the weather was poor we had problems, as jigsaws were really the only activity to occupy her. We persevered.

When autumn arrived, and with winter not far off, there were fewer outings for Elspeth. This was sad as she loved going out. Having said that, sometimes, when she had only been out a few minutes, she began saying certain things a lot more. Such as, *'Are we going back to your house?'* (meaning our house) or, *'Are we going back to your car?'* She did not want to stay out quite as much on many occasions. Five or six years ago, she was going out by herself for long walks in the countryside. How times had changed!

Elspeth stayed with carers until 5.00 pm when I took over for the evening and night shift—the day soon disappeared with all the jobs that had to be done to look after her and the house, coupled with the fact that there were a few hours of music work for the school's music company to do on the computer. Thank goodness for the music!

Tea was at about 6.00 pm. It took Elspeth a long time to begin eating her meal. I never knew why, as she still appeared to enjoy her food. She needed a lot of encouragement. Next was the bedtime routine. She would wander around upstairs for a while and never really go to sleep before I went to bed, which, if I was working, used to be anything up to midnight or even beyond. If any guests came in the evening before her bedtime, she would not know them. Gone were the days of putting on an annual Christmas or summer buffet for thirty or forty people. She no longer participated in entertaining others, having no idea what was happening. She always loved catering for large groups of friends here at home, and that would never happen again. I established a birthday barbecue for close friends, held on the nearest Saturday to August the 5th each year. She would never come into the garden to join in and see everybody, preferring to stay inside and do a jigsaw puzzle with a carer.

And so, my life revolved around her and being at home for two-thirds of the day unless I paid extra for someone to look after her. A 'wife-sitter', so to speak. There was, of course, no way she could ever be left alone. The duty of care fell to the carers and myself. She could not look after herself; she could not feed herself properly; she could not deal with her own personal hygiene; she could not even put herself to bed, and she was hardly sixty years old. Pick's disease was destroying her brain and shutting down its functions slowly but surely. I had read information about Pick's disease on virtually every website, and they all said the same thing: that we did not have many years left together. Maybe with a good diet, lots of brain stimulation and the best care possible, we could prove the websites wrong. We decided we would certainly try hard.

Here We Go Again

(First written at the end of September 2012)

We were still in limbo, waiting for financial decisions to be made which would deeply affect our family. I hadn't heard anything from Health for a few weeks. I was hoping that the current appeal was underway. Social Services had been in and out. Maybe we would know something about our financial situation before Christmas. It would be almost a year since all this business started.

The Sunday carer would arrive at 11.00 am on the dot. He would do a jigsaw with Elspeth as she continuously whispered *'Ellie Spelly'* in a rather mysterious voice. Quite ghostly! I think this name stemmed from when she was at school, and she was not a great 'speller'! Originally it was *'Ellie can't spelly'*! The carer and Elspeth would next go out for a drive to a nearby park. That meant a long walk if the weather held. One particular park was good for a variety of reasons, not the least important being that many farm animals were kept there for the public to view. Elspeth loved seeing these animals. Meanwhile, at home, I would set about preparing Sunday dinner. It's not difficult to become a better cook under these circumstances, thanks to recipe books and, of course, the internet. I always tried to cook at home, rather than buying ready prepared supermarket meals, to give Elspeth what I believed was a healthier diet. I must admit that occasionally, I did buy her favourite fish pie from the local supermarket. Being from the Grimsby and Cleethorpes area, she loved fish. I recall her telling me that as a student, she worked as a fish finger packer. Her co-workers, who were older regulars, were always telling her to be faster, as they needed to keep up their quota and would lose bonuses if they didn't reach certain targets! I also remember the marvellous fish pies her mother used to make when we visited, using the excellent haddock from Grimsby market. Grandpa always served Muscadet wine with it, and HP sauce was never missing from the table!

Going to the dentist was interesting. Elspeth was enrolled at a special dentist who was experienced at treating patients with dementia or mental disabilities. Once, to be safe, I did not give Elspeth a morning tablet as she was due for sedation before some serious work on her teeth. No food or drink for two hours before the appointment. The carer came with us, and when we arrived, as usual, she did not know where we were and kept asking, *'Are we going for a drive?'* She was given a small container of evil-looking green liquid, which she drank immediately. She then had anaesthetic cream put on the backs of both her hands so that a needle could be inserted to keep the supply of anaesthetic constant. After about three-quarters of an hour, she seemed calm, so we went into the dentist's room, where five staff members saw to her. The carer and I left them to it! She was having a filling, which took about forty-five minutes, together with taking out a dead root – the dentist thought she had swallowed the crown that was there before. The dental team was superb. Calmly and with good humour going about their business, an amazing team. At the end they gave her a cup of tea and accompanied us to the car in case she was still a bit wobbly! That afternoon we had been advised not to let her walk, so the carer took her on a short drive just so she could get out of the house. She went to bed at 7.30 pm, and that's when the slight problem began. She was not allowed a zopiclone sleeping tablet, and the result was she didn't sleep a wink all night. Unfortunately, she spent the whole night wanting to get out of bed. I didn't let her do this, so she turned her attention to poking and scratching me. She used to feel for a rough piece of skin and scratch it till it came away (if I didn't try to stop her)! The more I attempted to keep her away, the more she tried to scratch. It was out of the question to go and sleep in another room, as I did not know how she might behave with no one there to keep an eye on her. I saw every hour through until she got up at the usual time of 7.00 am. I had to make sure she was ready for the 9.00 am carer's visit. I was shattered but Elspeth seemed no different to usual! Off she went enthusiastically for her morning outing. I sat down in an armchair after doing a few jobs and had a nap. I would have been able to manage better if it wasn't for one of my gout attacks on my left foot instep and big toe. Rather limiting, and those people who suffer from this affliction will know exactly what I mean. It would subside in a few days, but it made life difficult. I certainly made sure that Elspeth took all necessary tablets that night!

One More Step

(First written in April 2013)

Another important matter had now been resolved for the time being, and that was finances. Funding for Elspeth's care package had been sorted out. Even though the result was not particularly good for us, at least we knew where we stood. The situation was that the NHS would fund twenty-two hours out of the fifty-eight hours (as it was by now) of care a week that Elspeth needed. The cost of the whole package was well over £40,000 p/a. Social Services would contribute around £7000 towards this, so we had to find the rest. We would naturally use Elspeth's state pension and Disability Living Allowance (DLA) – soon to become Personal Independence Payment (PIP), together with any savings she had, which amounted to an ISA and a bond, both of which she had carefully saved to be given to our daughters in later life. We did know that when her savings dropped below the level of £23,500, we could receive more help with our payments.

At that time, the Alzheimer's Society let it be known that due to funding difficulties, their Outreach service might need to charge clients later in the year. This meant we would have to drop their input, losing the six hours a week we were allotted. There would be no way we could afford up to (possibly) an extra £5000 p/a to keep Outreach. This was extremely sad, as the AS was the first agency to help Elspeth, what seemed like a lifetime ago now. The carers from this marvellous, professional institution were simply terrific at all times.

Now we had to wait for the next big meeting to see if we could convince the NHS that Elspeth's behavioural needs were 'severe' rather than, in their view, 'high'. I struggled to understand how her behaviour had *improved* over the years when it was clearly so much worse. I didn't think, however, that we would win, as I couldn't see them changing their mind and granting us full funding again. It turned out that way.

I had to spend most of my time at home – a kind of 'imposed isolation' -unless a carer or someone else was with Elspeth. Included in her package was money for some hours a year of evening cover, but this dwindled quickly as I was involved with music concerts for children and young people on three or four evenings a year. I needed to keep this work going to give me something else to think about. Otherwise, life was limited to staying at home and looking after Elspeth, although this was unquestionably my priority.

I worked with a Youth Theatre (and still do), for which I wrote the music for several productions, ran the choir, and gave concerts at the local junior school. I would have had to use most of any evening allowance for this, had my daughters not helped me out by looking after their mother. Alice was singing for a Sheffield group at the time, giving many concerts in Sheffield and beyond, and I wanted very much to hear her and them perform. By the time we'd had a couple of evening birthday meals out in the year, there wasn't much left in the kitty!

Meanwhile, Elspeth was about the same. Up at 7.00 am every day, breakfast and jigsaws till the carer came at 9.00 am. Dressing in the morning was becoming even more difficult, as she had completely forgotten how to do this. She would walk straight past the bathroom, asking if she was going back to bed. I had to turn her round and aim her in the right direction! She had to be guided in all the normal 'morning routine' activities. If I didn't watch her, she would go back to bed, sometimes putting her nightie over her day clothes. Carers would take her out after the jigsaw, but bad weather, especially snow, put a stop to that. Searching for any new activity which might interest her, we discovered she would thread beads or colour in patterns for quite a while. It is heartbreaking to remember what a fine artist she was – our house still has a lot of her pictures displayed on the walls. (I enjoyed going into her art college folder and selecting pictures to frame and hang). Now, she was reduced to 'colouring in'. The bead activity came to an abrupt end when she started putting the beads into her mouth! We couldn't allow that to go on.

Elspeth had been shouting *'Ellie Spelly'* on her walks for most of the time during the outing. You could hear her in the distance. You also knew when she had arrived back home because of the noise. Often on return, she would need changing because of an 'accident'. Tea and bed followed the afternoon walks. She still ate everything placed in front of her. In bed, she would lie staring into space for two or three hours. If she did doze off, I had to wake her up when I gave her a sleeping tablet at about 10.00 pm! If I was lucky, she would then sleep till 7.00 am. If I was unlucky, she would wake at 3.00 am, put all the lights on, go to the bathroom and, turn on taps, then leave them on and come back to bed, muttering. I needed to get up and turn everything off.

In order to look after Elspeth's finances, as she was not able to do so, I had to have Power of Attorney. Unfortunately, she was not able to sign any documents because of her lack of cognition, so I had to apply to the courts through our solicitors, which cost a lot of money - more money. Savings were disappearing fast! I also had to become her Deputy through the Office of the Public Guardian, and I was regularly checked to make sure I was looking after her interests properly. There was a lengthy annual report to fill in. It was expensive being a Deputy since after massive solicitor's fees for POA, there was £320 p/a to pay for the privilege, plus another £250 p/a for a bond to cover her savings.

More and More

(First written at the end of January 2014)

2014 was going to be an interesting year. Much would happen over the next twelve months. To understand the situation, you needed to be with Elspeth to see what was happening to her. People still said to me, 'Does she ask about *this*/ laugh about *that*/ show a reaction to *the other*?' The answer was 'No!' none of this happened, and it hadn't happened for a long time. Not many people (except carers and hospital visitors – lots of them) came to our house now, so it meant that few really understood the nature of this illness. If, by chance, anyone else popped in, they would find her behaviour unusual, to say the least – especially if they had known her when she was 'well'. She had now lost much of her interest in jigsaws, so activities were limited, and of course, there was no conversation. Not long ago, she would have 'jigsawed' by herself for hours. She still spent some time with jigsaw puzzles, but only if someone sat with her and stopped her from standing up and walking around. Happily, the jigsaws had served a very useful purpose for three years. She would, however, sit and 'paint' if someone was sitting with her. Carers would draw the outline of a shape, and Elspeth would fill it in with block colour. She applied paint very carefully, up to the edges of the shape and not over. One or two carers who watched her even found that her techniques taught them something new, helping them to improve their own artistic skills. It was, however, a far cry from the beautiful pictures she used to create when she was younger.

I am sure Elspeth also enjoyed 'Aquapainting' - simply brushing water onto an invisible picture which then magically appeared. This was, in fact, a very useful occupation, which she took to immediately. There were many different subjects, with five pictures in a pack, all geared towards those with dementia, ranging from Transport to Farm Animals, Birds, Flowers and Seaside etc. I would highly recommend this as a dementia activity.

Elspeth didn't sit still for long now. She had started walking endlessly from the kitchen to the front room and back again. Then to the front door and back again. She always tried the handles, only to find that the doors were locked – this was on purpose, as she had taken to 'escaping' from the house whenever she could. Four times in the past, she had been seen walking down the road, twice in her dressing gown, once wearing a wet-hair 'turban' and slippers and once with no trousers on. Luckily, on that occasion, she was wearing a long cardigan. She had also locked carers in the garage three times when they had gone in there to turn off the toilet light! Fortunately, I was there to unlock the door. It wasn't that she meant to lock them out; she just wanted to lock the door. We really had to be on our guard to watch her the whole time.

In the evenings, when Elspeth went to bed, she tended to get up again and walk to the toilet more than before. Since she flooded the kitchen by not turning the taps off, I had to put locks on the bathroom and toilet doors. We used to let her into the toilet a couple of times, although her many visits rarely resulted in her doing anything except using up vast quantities of toilet paper and increasing the water bill! Sitting in the front room, I used to hear her footsteps on the bedroom floor through the ceiling. You can imagine that after a while, it became very distracting. If I tried to put her to bed, she would be up again very quickly. When I did go to bed she would start running her hand over my head, or try to find a bit of rough skin and scratch it! Not good when you're tired, but I expect she just wanted to feel that someone was there. I often ended up at the edge of my side of the bed, not daring to go to another room in case she did anything dangerous and I wasn't aware of it. Anyway, since our old mattress was so ancient and had body-shaped dents in it, I had invested in a comfy new mattress and quilt, and I wasn't going to be deprived of those!

Continence was becoming more of a problem and not very pleasant. Sometimes, the carers changed her twice a day, and I did a third change in the evening. She had a habit of 'performing' whilst walking around. The NHS Continence Team had allocated us three pairs of pants a day, which was very helpful. Highest absorbency, naturally.

We continued to visit the excellent specialist dentist. I thought I had secured a house visit one day, but her schedule was too heavy on the day I had booked, so a carer and I took Elspeth to the surgery. All was well, though it was a bit of a fight to keep her in the chair. We didn't have to sedate her this time. I had also arranged a visit from the mobile opticians, as Elspeth had been putting everyone's spectacles on! She appeared not to be seeing too well from one side. Two pleasant chaps came to us, but they hadn't got a great deal of knowledge about her illness. The first thing they said was, *'Can you read out what this card says?'* There was no reaction from Elspeth. Anyway, we managed to keep her still whilst the opticians had a good look, and we ordered a pair of glasses for her, which actually looked quite nice. I was not convinced that she needed them, but I think they may have helped with close observation at the table.

We continued to spend Elspeth's money every month on her care fees. On average, the cost was around £2000, £400 of which was from DLA or PIP. Her state pension and savings paid the rest. I worried about what might happen when her reserves ran out and I still wasn't sure whether the Council would increase their contribution. If her money supply dried up, the last thing I wanted to do was reduce her care package or, even worse, take on the role of a full-time carer. I would have to wait and see how events turned out.

I wasn't expecting to have such a limited life at this point, having to spend most of my time at home being a carer for all those hours a week, but there would be others who were in the same boat, and I had a strong empathy with them. I felt extremely fortunate to be able to work for the music company from home and to have two hours a week working with children up at the local school. Besides this, having a carer on a Sunday meant I could keep my work going with young people at Wentworth Youth Theatre. It was very difficult to go out even for a simple pub meal, and I knew we would never be able to go on holiday together again, the last one being a weekend at Robin Hood's Bay with friends a few years earlier. That was fraught with difficulties, in particular, keeping an eye on Elspeth. (An interesting incident from that short break was that she wore a pair of shoes with the soles coming away and flapping about. She refused to let us change them. When she had gone to bed on the first night, we threw them into the bin and put out a new pair I had taken with us in anticipation of being able to exchange them for the faulty pair. The next day, Elspeth did not notice at all that she was wearing a different pair of shoes!)

I continued to think and worry about whether NHS/Social Services would withdraw any funding – that would put a spanner in the works, as we could not afford to pay any more. I thought back to Elspeth being fully funded and how, as far as finance was concerned, there was little stress over money in those days. I was not a happy bunny and was getting somewhat fed up with the way things were going. Elspeth had become very vague, having to be guided in most directions and constantly watched. As you know, Pick's probably has a span of around two to twelve years. Our aim had always been and would always be to do as much as possible for her and for as long as possible. 'Non Deficere'!

Interestingly, the word 'home', as in residential care, is now being mentioned in conversations with various parties. I discussed this with our most excellent CPN. During her time with us, this lady provided us with magnificent help and advice, for which I shall be eternally grateful. It would all depend on what help we would receive with costs. It would be a massive relief to me to have this weight taken away, but there was still a lot of me that said Elspeth seemed happy here at home, and that is where she must stay until the last possible moment. I believed that she still recognised her surroundings (maybe), though I wasn't sure how long that would last. Anyway, her interests would always come first. I would look into the home idea, where she could be properly looked after twenty-four hours a day by caring staff. I might even get a decent sleep!

Extracts From a Newsletter To Friends and Family

(Sent 25th May 2014)

Morning All,

Carer just arrived so that's Elspeth being looked after till bathtime at 6.00 pm. The weather is not too good today, but they will still go out with a big umbrella!

As you will be expecting, Elspeth's condition slowly and inevitably deteriorates. She is sitting with Bob, the carer, now doing a jigsaw before they go out. If he wasn't there, she would immediately stand up and begin walking from front to back door, trying the handles and laughing. Not very good when I am trying to write songs here at the computer. Wish she'd tell us the joke because it seems really funny! She loves going out but is not always keen on the walking bit. It's good when she has a long walk as that makes her tired, and hopefully, she sleeps better. She eats very well – and healthily. She has put on a lot of weight, but I am told that could be the pills she has to take.

One good thing is that she will now watch a bit of TV, though she hasn't a clue what is going on. I think she likes the bright colours of the Disney Channel – she may sit for half an hour before getting up to walk around. The other night the girls were both here and they wanted the film 'Frozen' on Box Office. Elspeth watched the whole movie all the way through for ninety minutes, which was quite remarkable. I have put a small TV up in the bedroom, hoping it might keep her occupied when she goes to bed. I think the idea has partially worked, but she still wanders to the loo regularly, although she does not need to. I think I told you we now lock the bathroom door in the evenings since she left the taps on and blew the main fuse one fateful Saturday night. She has to be guided all over the place, bathed and dressed (mostly), but she eats by herself, that is, if someone is sitting with her and helping. Of course, she has no conversation and often talks gibberish or laughs in a weird way. She is difficult to look after and must still be closely watched at all times. One mistake, and she would be off down the road. A glass of red wine carelessly left out, and she would drink it down fast and be sick, as happened recently.

Continence is dreadful, but the less said about that, the better. Our excellent CPN has been ill, so we have not seen anyone from that department for a while, including the consultant who is overseeing Elspeth's case. The nurse used to visit every month or so for five or six years. I shall have to contact them soon, as I am considering reducing the paid care hours, and I need to discuss that! It seems that I sit here at home working on the computer, particularly in the mornings, while carers sit in the other room doing jigsaws or watching TV, which is all they can do. I reckon if they weren't there, Elspeth would walk, but I could keep half an eye on her whilst working and save about £6k a year. We have already spent about £25k of Elspeth's money in the last two years on care, plus £10k DLA, and I am starting to feel as if I don't want to part with lots more money. I want to pass as much as possible on to the girls. Looks like a lump of my state pension (I am so old!), which begins in August, will have to go towards fees, as I can't keep going to savings accounts.

The only answer is to reduce hours, and I hope the NHS continues to fund their twenty-two hours a week. I am afraid we are witnessing Elspeth slowly fading away, which is very sad. I do not know what the situation will be like, even by Christmas, or even if she will be in a home. Where might the money come from for that?

Hope you are all well! I'm ok – just wish these figures and money signs would stop going around in my head! Ha ha!

Love from,

Ian, Elspeth, and the very grown-up Catriona and Alice.

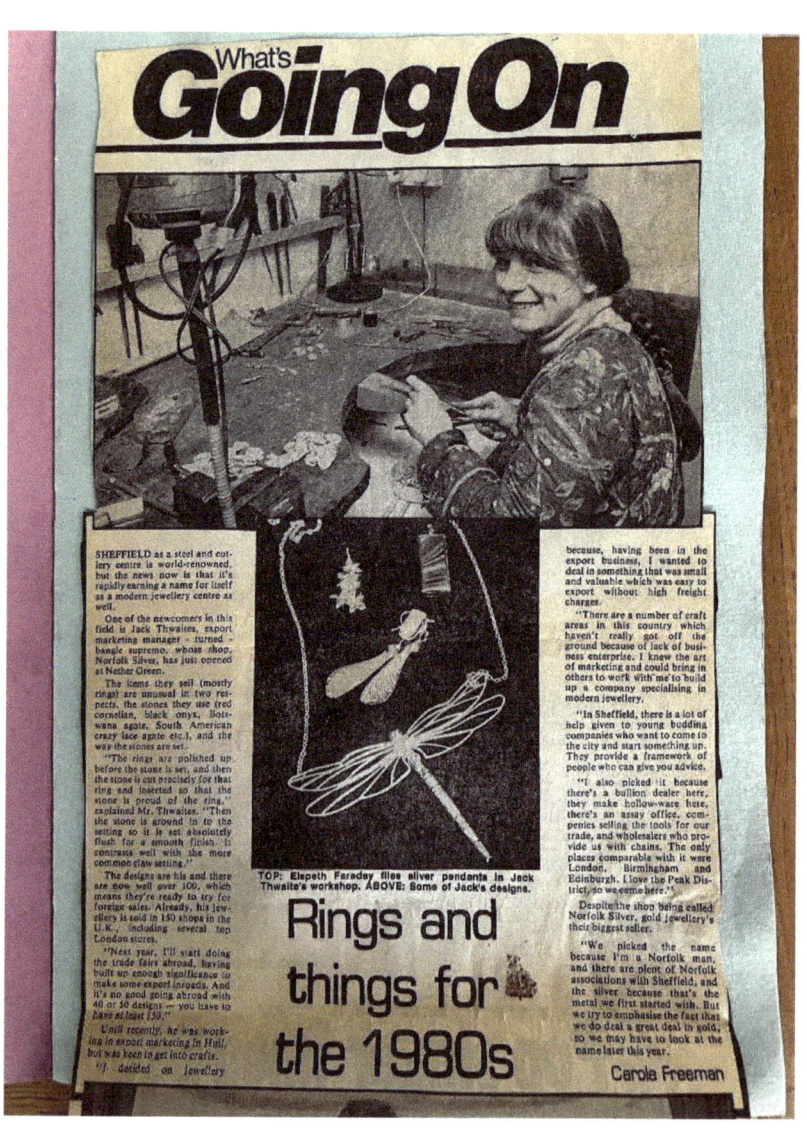

A newspaper cutting showing Elspeth at work

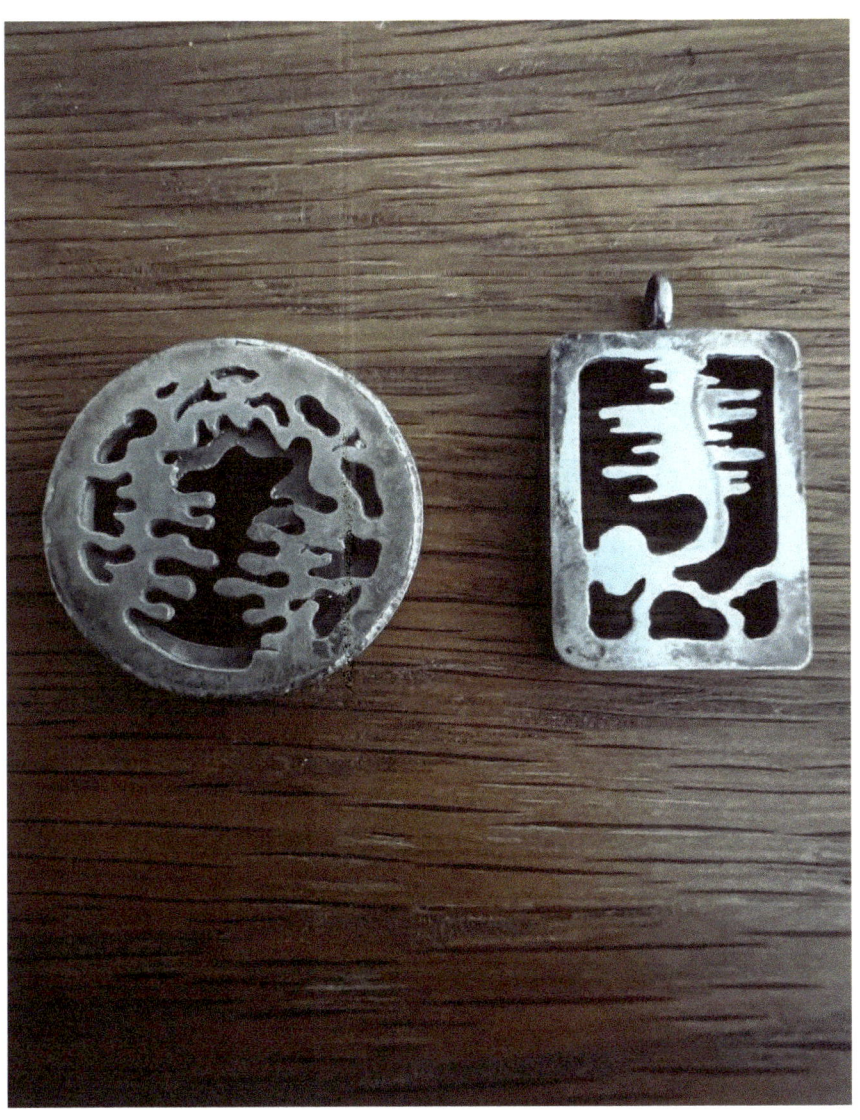

Unpolished silver jewellery, cut out and ready for the next stage

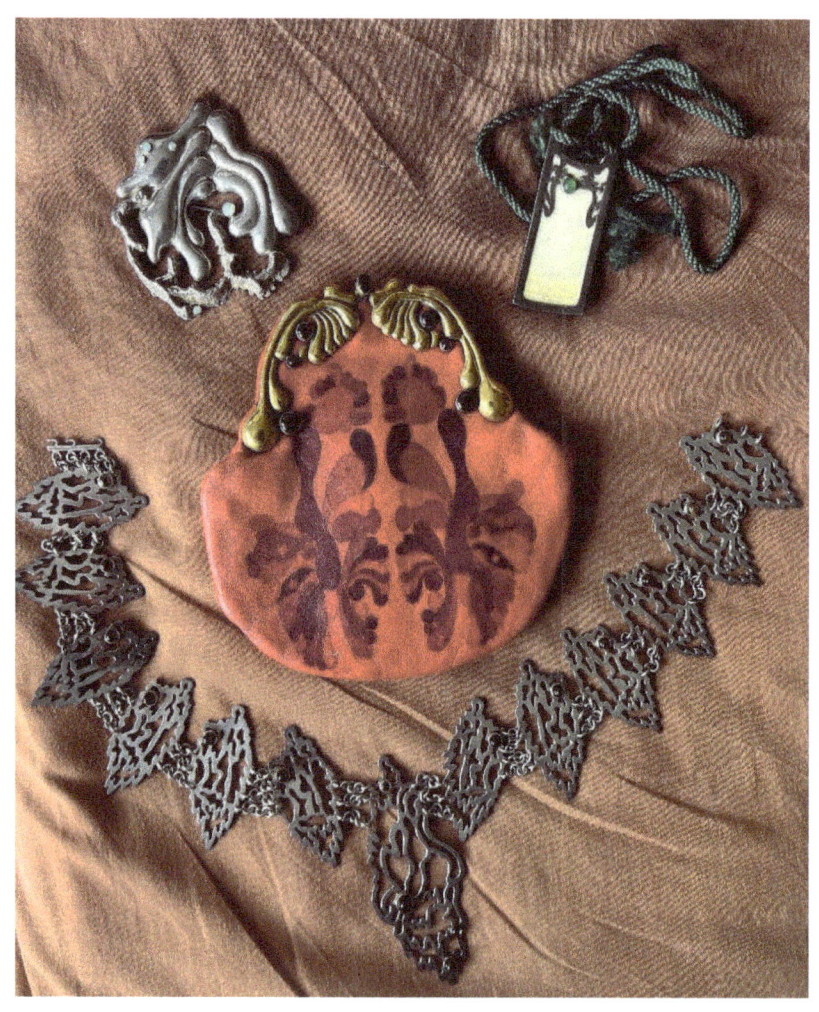

Some of Elspeth's exhibition jewellery from her college finals

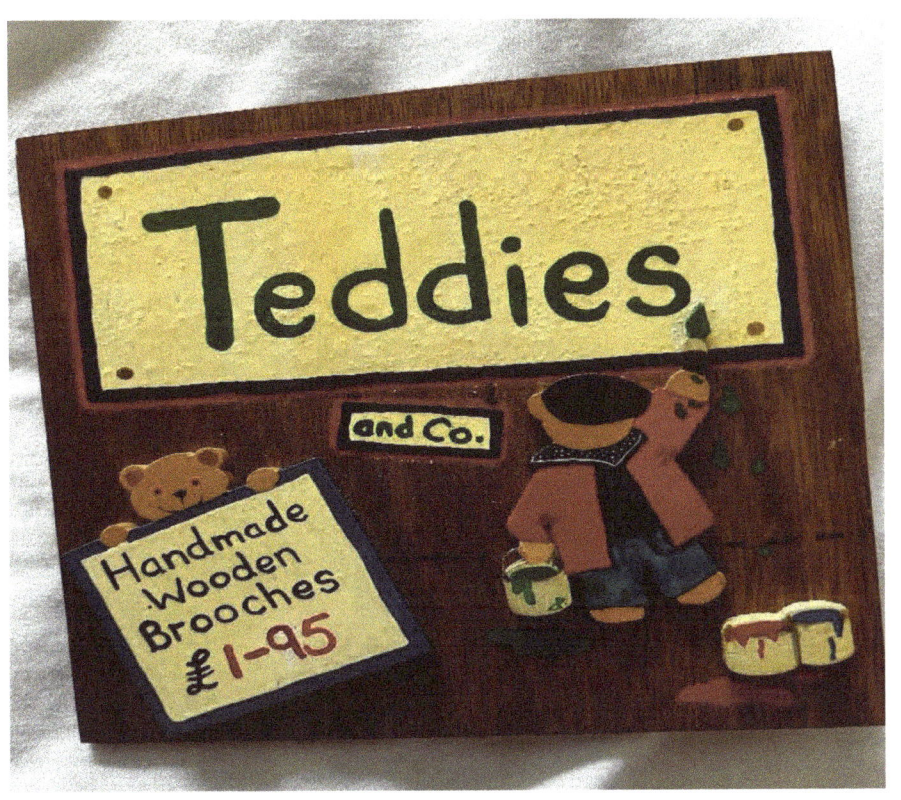

Teddies for sale!

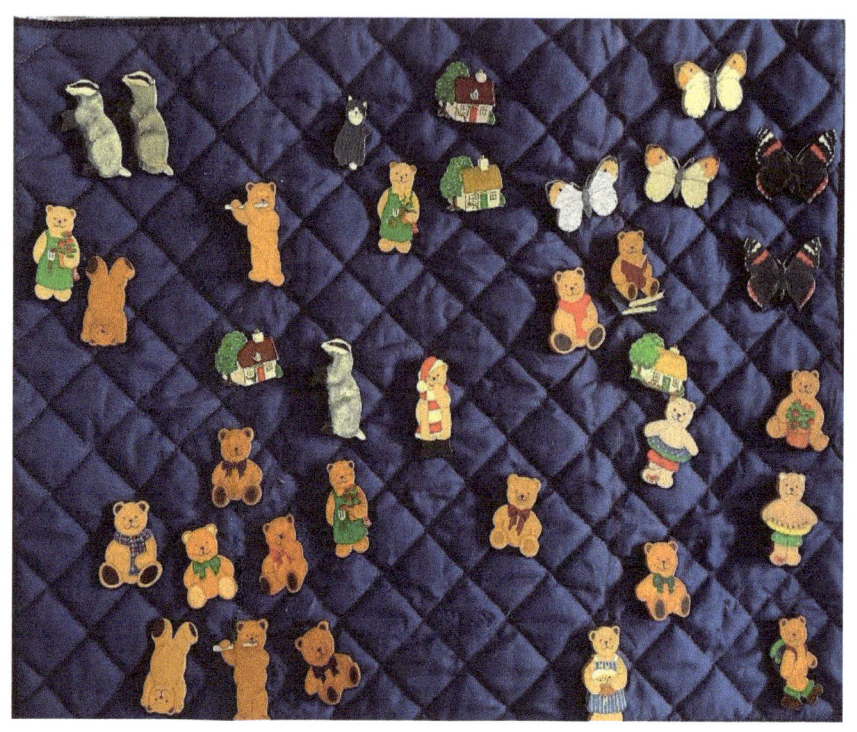

Different hand-made wooden badges

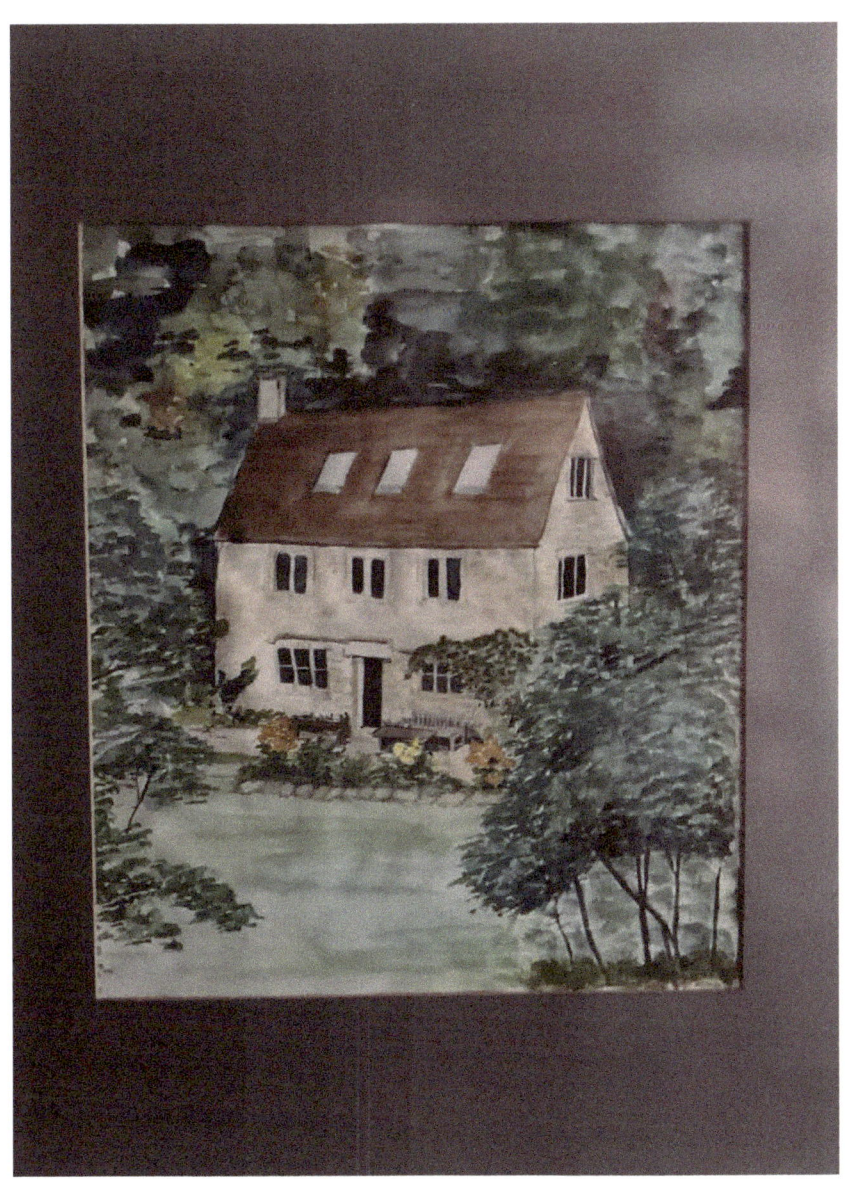

A holiday cottage drawn from a photo

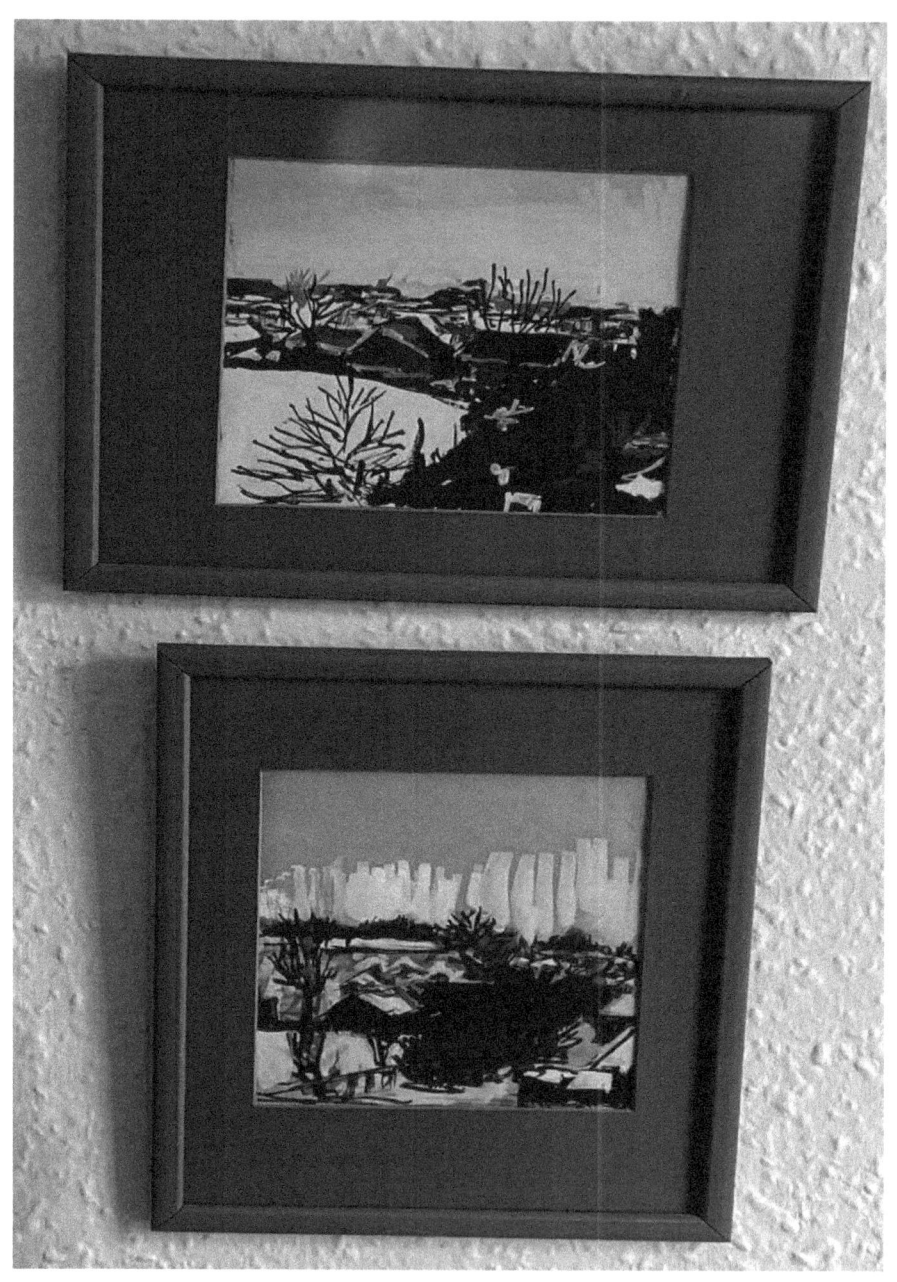

Snow scenes

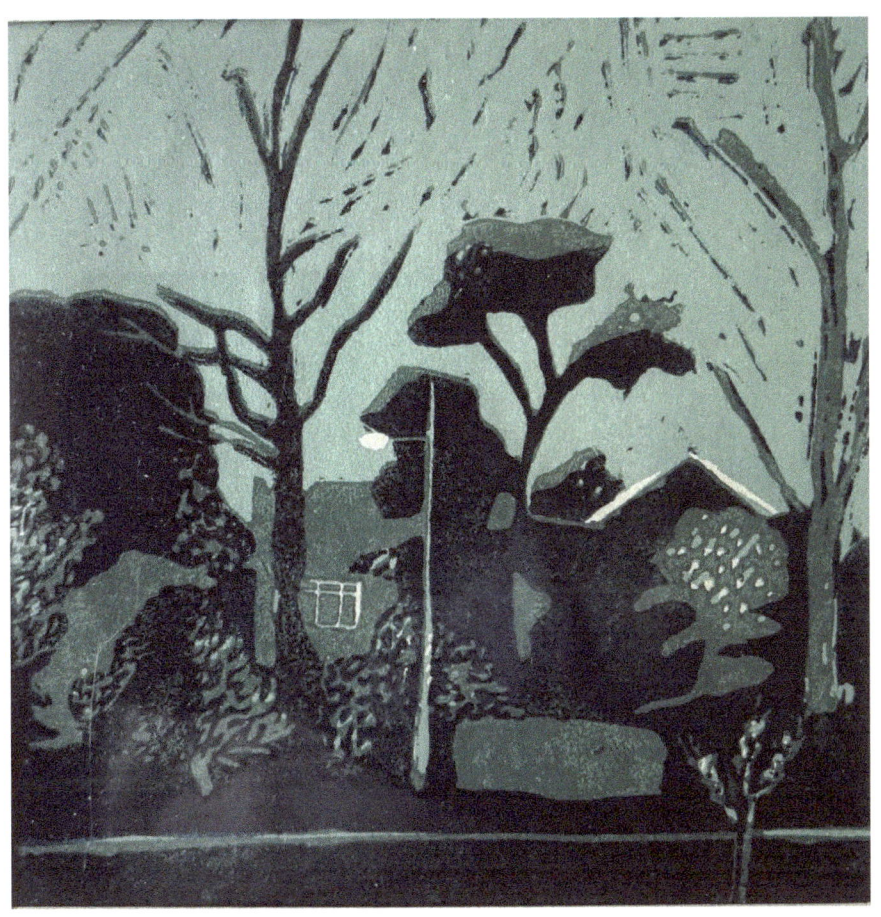

Green houses!

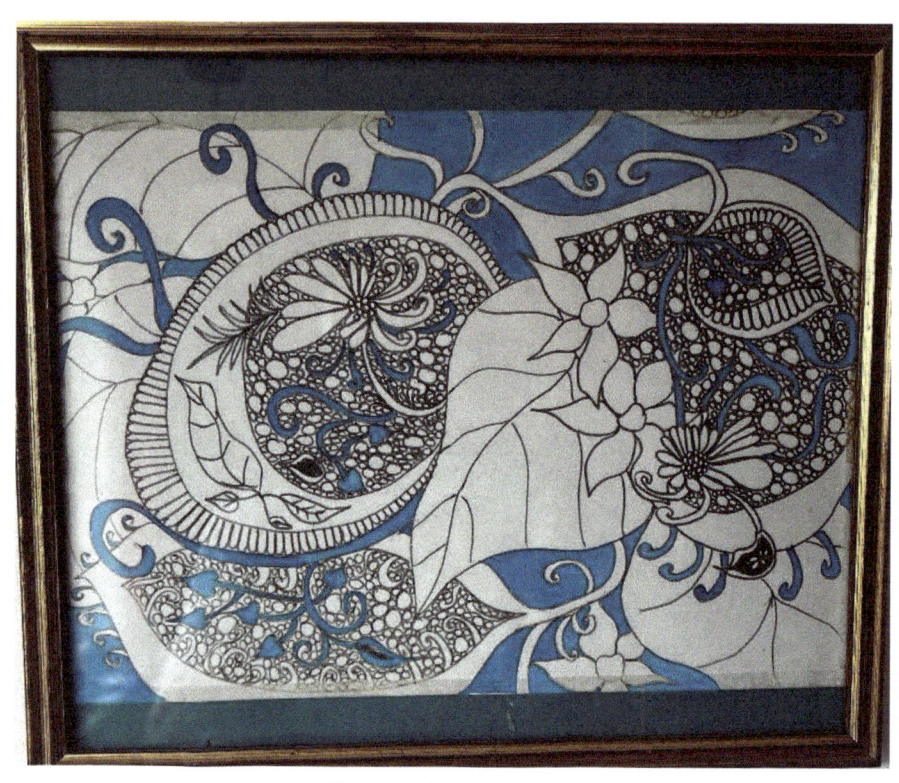

Interesting patterns

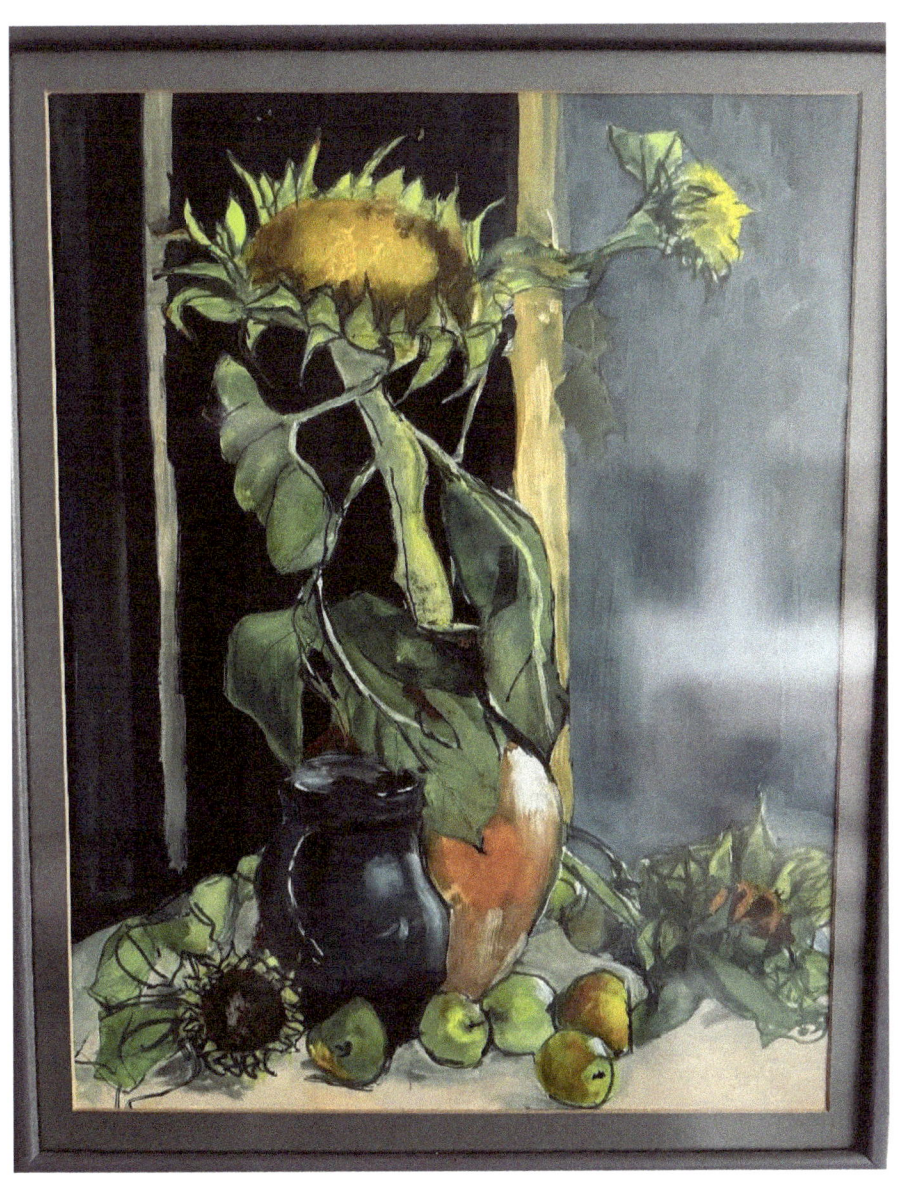

Sunflowers

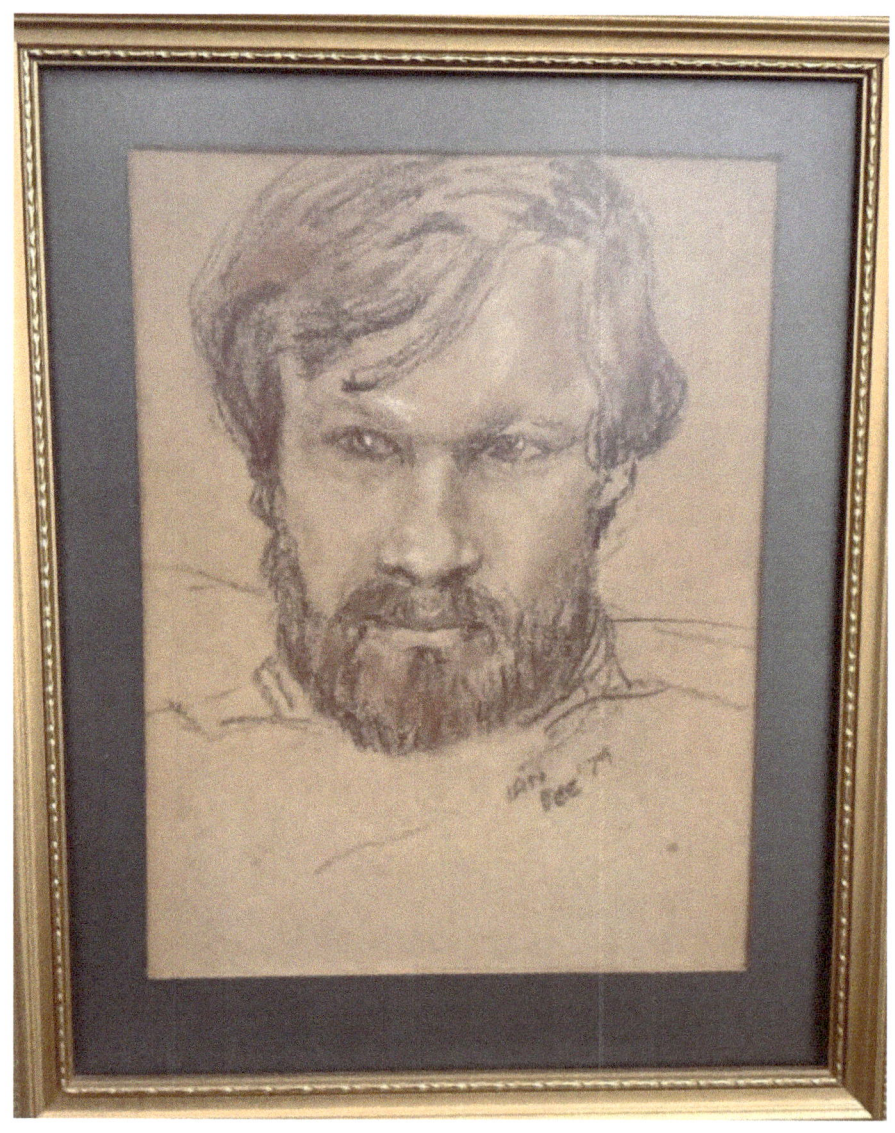

Elspeth's drawing of Ian in 1979

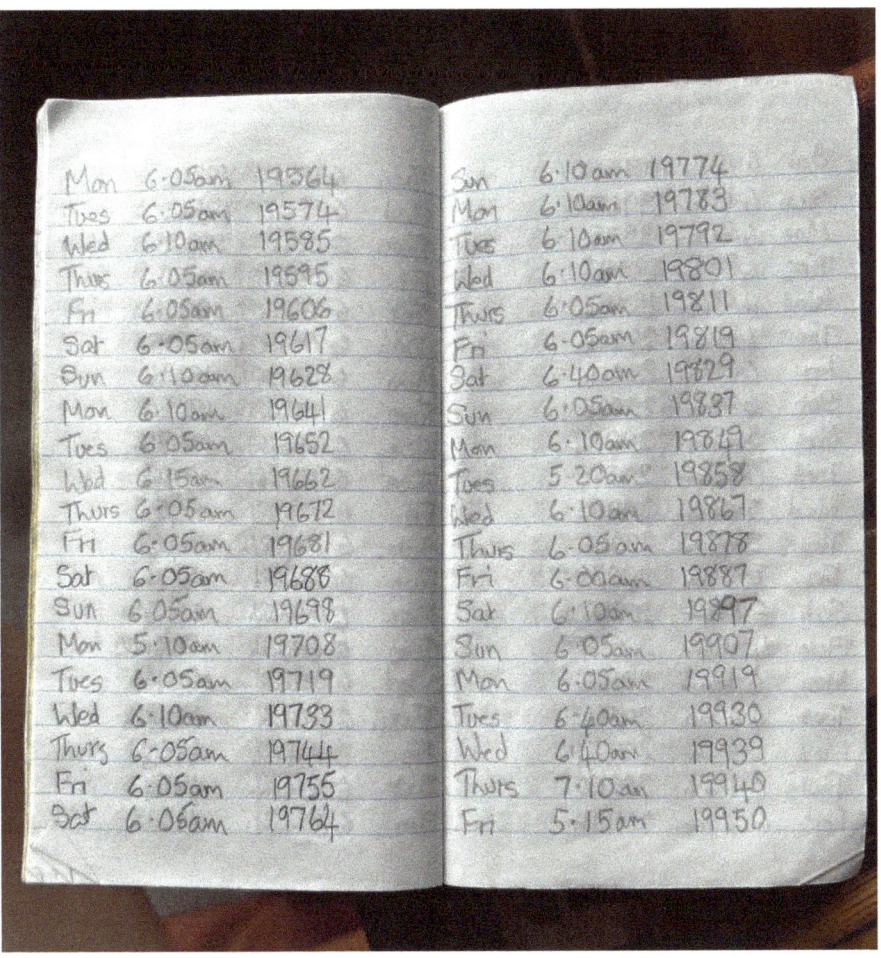

Two of many pages of meter readings

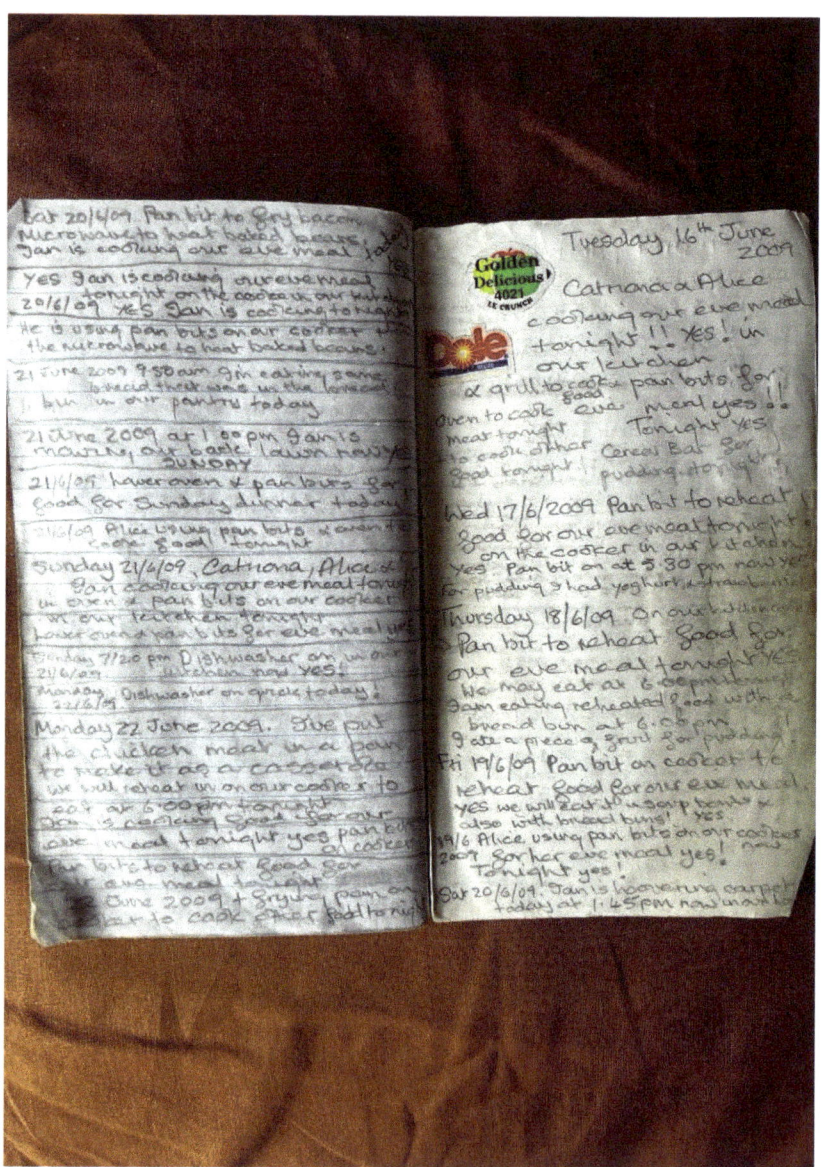

An example of Elspeth's diary entries

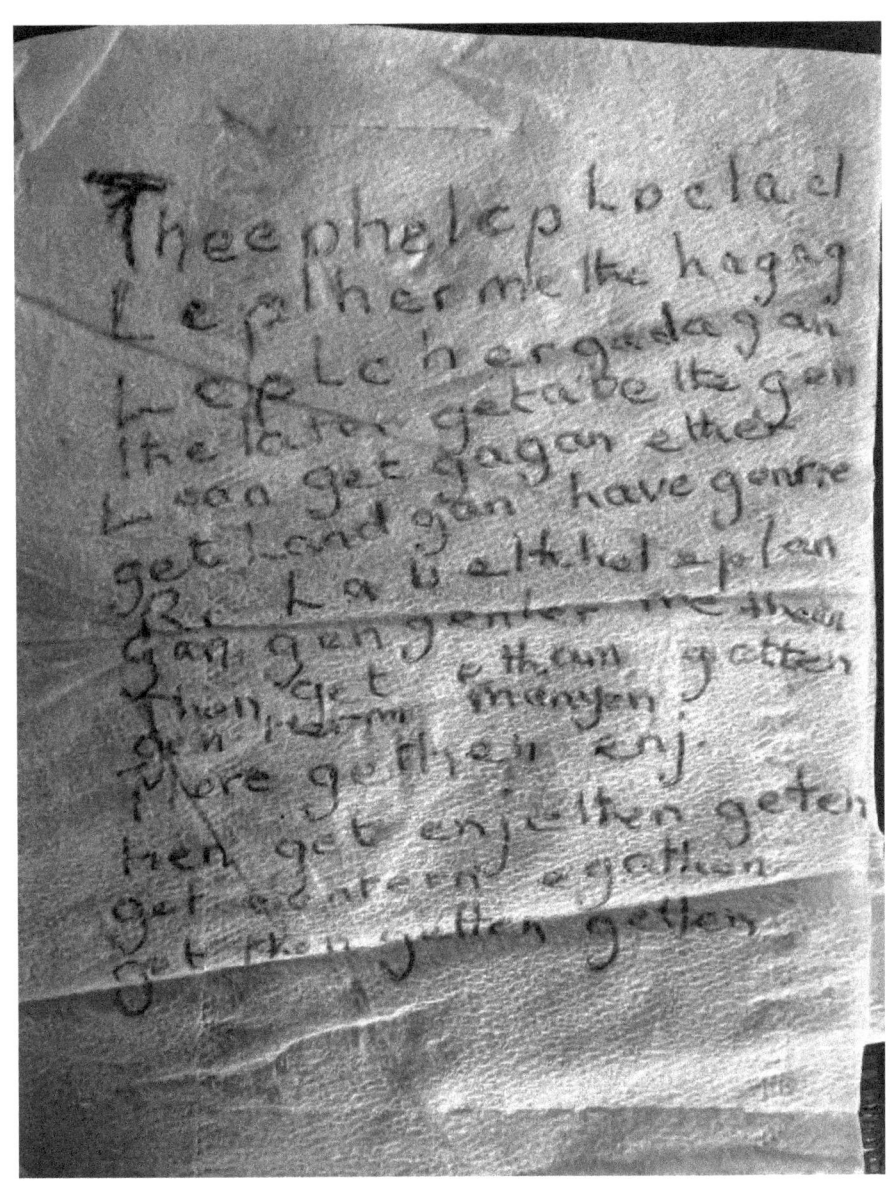

A further example of Elspeth's strange writings

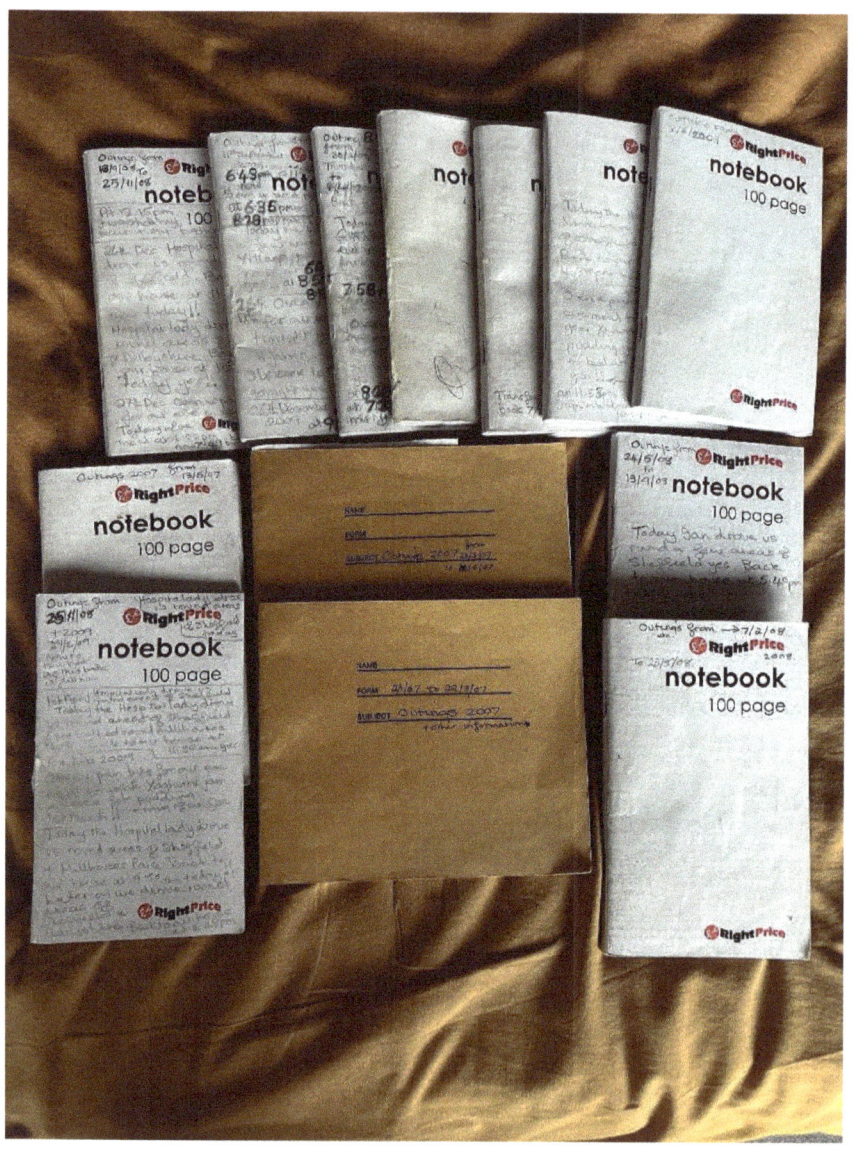

Some of Elspeth's many diaries, each filled with day by day accounts of her outings

Wedding Photos 1976

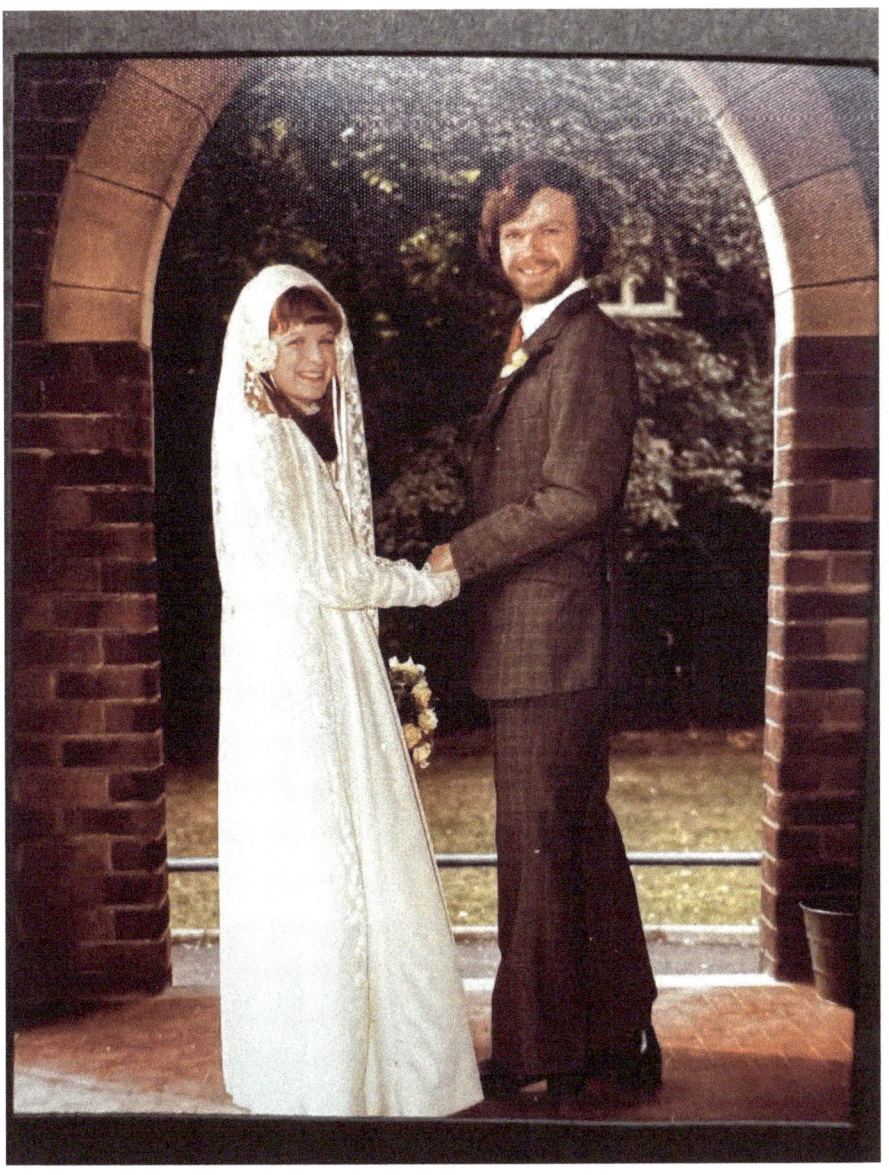

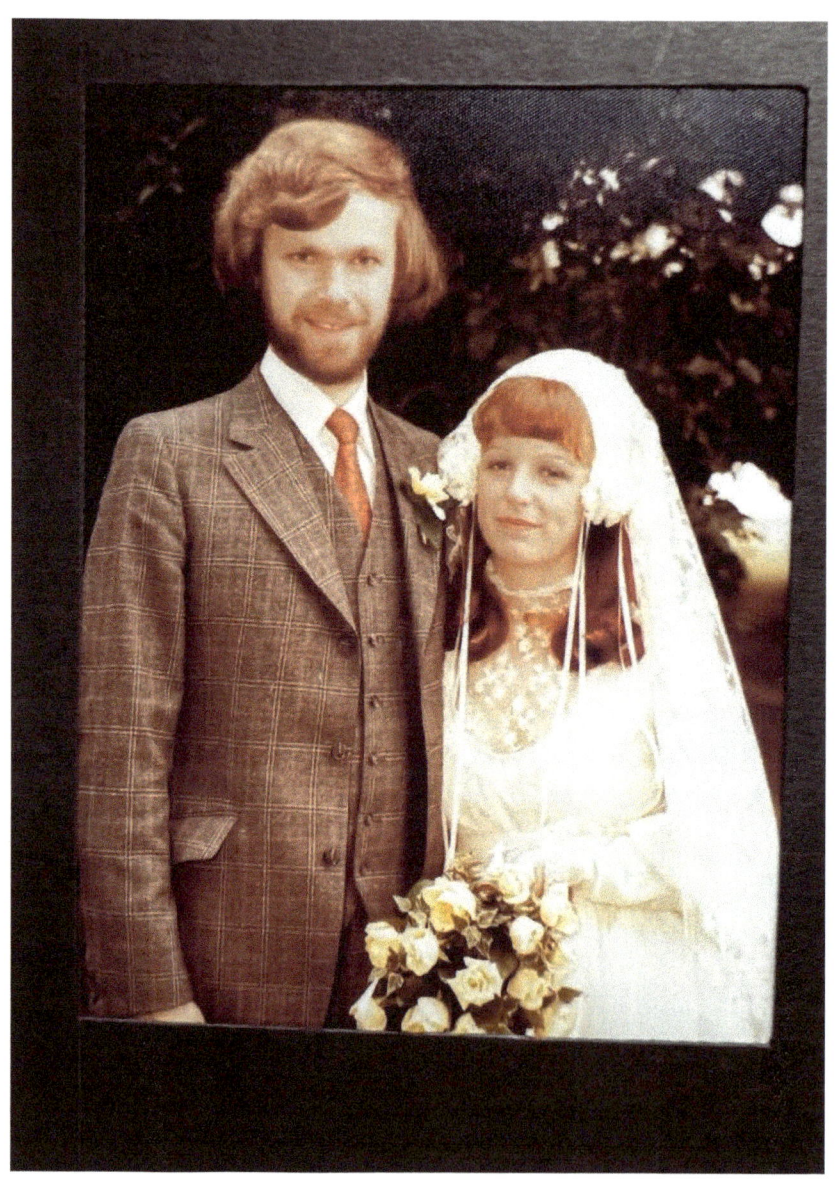

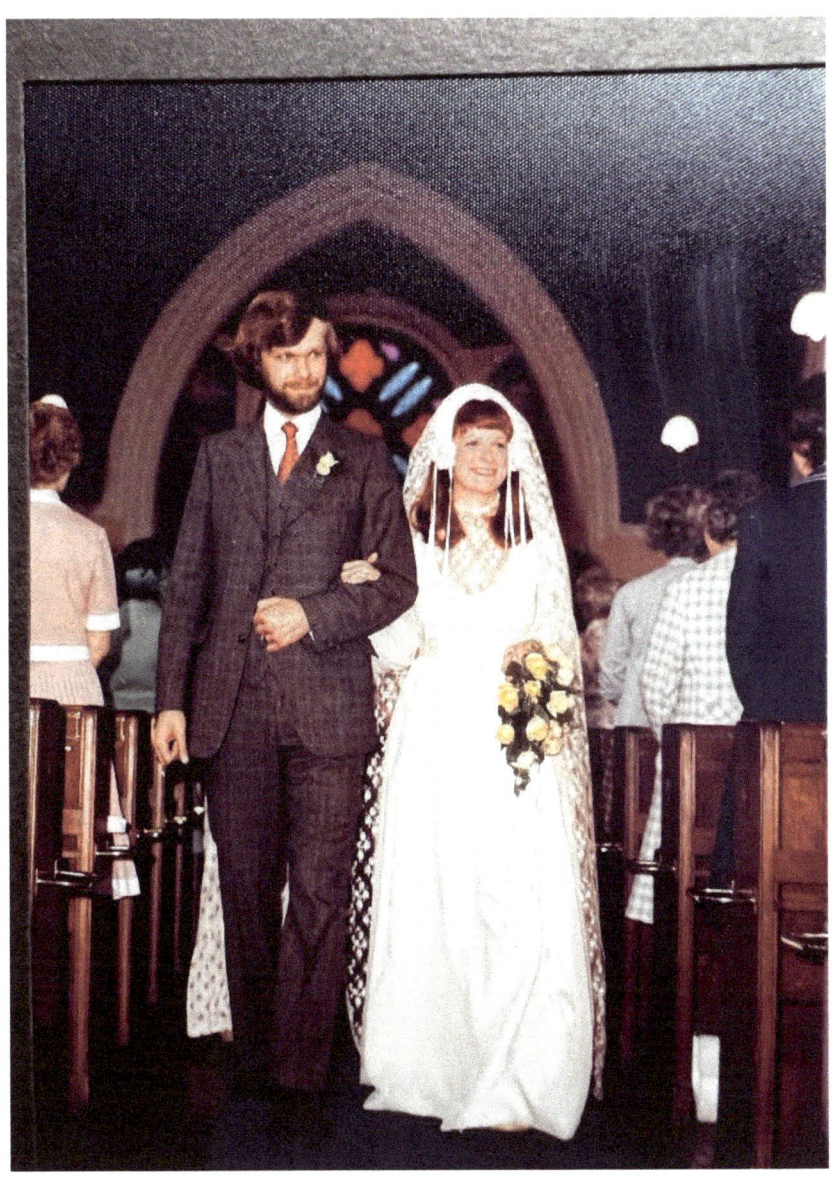

Up to Date

(Written 17th August 2014)

Recently, Elspeth had twice made a bid for freedom. Fortunately, she had only managed to reach the gateway on our drive before I was able to guide her back inside. This had happened at the change-over time for carers and had been my fault for not locking the doors immediately. It was so easy to show someone into the house and take your eyes off her for a few seconds. During that brief time, she was off out of the house! I think somewhere in her head, there was a vague memory of past walks and a desire to hit the open road again. Or maybe she just wanted to get away from everyone. We had to tighten up in this area as we did not want any disasters.

One Sunday, Elspeth got out of bed at about 7.30 am and headed to the toilet. We had been through a pretty rough night, so I was half asleep. I remember hearing the toilet flush and then the bathroom tap being turned on. I was conscious of her coming back to bed. I always get up to check things out, but that morning, I didn't. It must have been ten minutes later when I heard loud dripping sounds coming from the bathroom and the ominous noise of the water tank filling in the loft. I jumped out of bed to find the bathroom floor flooded. Hot water was pouring over the side of the sink. The plug was still in. I turned the tap off and pulled the plug out before mopping the floor with any available towels. I remember how nice and warm those tiles felt as I stood on them with bare feet. Downstairs, the kitchen was flooded, and water had once again cascaded down through the ceiling light. I threw the switch on the relevant fuse and began the great kitchen 'mop-up'. Elspeth stayed in bed during all this, which was a help. The following day, the electrician came to check everything out, and although there was still a little water in the light fitting, he dealt with that, and we were given the all-clear. Since that day, the bathroom door was locked in the evenings, which, although inconvenient, at least stopped the same thing from happening again.

Elspeth always wore the gold ring that she had made for our wedding. Besides my wedding ring, I also used to wear a signet ring on another finger. This had been a twenty-first birthday present from my mum. Elspeth had cut that ring off me some years previously (when she was well!) because the finger on which I wore it had become a lot wider than it used to be! Both the finger and the knuckle had become swollen and numb. My wedding ring finger was going the same way, and that ring had to come off sometime later. We tried all the tricks of the trade to remove the signet ring, but nothing worked. Being a jeweller, she had a saw with a tiny-toothed blade, so I went with her, apprehensively, into the garage, where she reversed the blade and put a thin piece of cardboard between the ring and my finger. In about five minutes, the job was done, and off came the ring, leaving me with my finger still intact and only a small blister. It was a relief in more ways than one! She put the ring away in a box somewhere, and I didn't find it for ages.

Going back to Elspeth's ring, it seemed that the same thing was happening to her ring finger. The girls and I tried soap, butter, the string trick and other clever ideas, but with no result. We were going to have to take her to the hospital when, after one Sunday dinner, Alice, my younger daughter, tried olive oil - and it worked! Although having to remove the ring after thirty-five years was sad, the painless 'operation' had to be carried out. It did not seem to bother Elspeth, who just accepted it. As mentioned earlier, Alice now looks after her mother's engagement and wedding rings and wears them on special occasions, which makes me happy. I think she particularly likes the engagement ring and the way the three opals flash in different colours when light hits them.

I was with Elspeth more than anyone, and her constant deterioration was apparent. She would not wash herself in the morning unless I stood by her and gave her the flannel. She would not brush her teeth unless I put toothpaste on the brush and handed it to her. She often wandered into the toilet for a few seconds and then came straight out again. I had taken the inside bolt off the door so she could not lock herself in. Someone also had to pull her pants down before she remembered what to do. All this meant that she had to be cleaned up two or three times a day, and her many baths had become essential. She quietly allowed all this to happen, whether it was with male or female carers. She didn't say much, as she was starting to lose the ability to speak coherently. She often whispered the words *'spee mee'*, which was a corruption of *'eve meal'*. She was going through a period of shortening words for some reason – our road, Devonshire Road, became *'Dev Road'*. *'Spee mee'* could often be heard if she woke during the night. At the time, this was a danger sign, which would usually be followed by her grabbing my arm and attempting to scratch. Sleep was difficult. By now, she had forgotten how to dress herself in the mornings, and this had to be done for her before she headed downstairs. Often, after being dressed in 'clean everything' at 8.30 am, she would need changing again before the carer came at 9.00 am. It was only fair to Elspeth and the carer that I did this before the arrival of the carer rather than leave it for their first job.

I had an idea that I wanted to lower the costs for care, paid for by Elspeth, out of her savings. As these were disappearing fast, I was prepared to cope with a few more hours a week at home, so I put some thought into a new timetable for the care agency jointly funded by Elspeth and the Council. I talked to the management and gave them a copy of my proposals. I had a visit from the Social Services, and I brought this subject up. It could be that if I reduced hours with the agency then it was possible that Continuing Health would follow suit and reduce their hours. As I was not sure about this, and it would have made life impossible here, I scrapped the idea. We very much needed the care, especially in the afternoons. In the next couple of years Elspeth's savings would be down to the threshold. £19240 is a huge amount of money to find over a year, even though it is reduced by a little over £5000 due to her DLA payment. It was all about money or lack of it! I contacted Sheffield Council regarding a financial assessment for Elspeth. I had several questions to ask, but I basically wanted to know when there would be more help available with payments. After sending me a letter to arrange a visit, I had a phone call on the morning of the visit to say they would not be coming until Elspeth's finances dropped to £23,500. Think again, Ian!

I mentioned earlier about the possibility of having to do without the services of the Alzheimer's Society, as there was a chance they would have to charge clients for Outreach. It was good news to hear that the Society had secured funding for another year at least. I would have found it very hard to be without their excellent input. There would be a charge for all mileage when Elspeth was taken out, but that would be about £30 per month. That seemed a highly acceptable price to pay for what they did for Elspeth. I hoped that we would hear similar news the following year.

Around this time, Elspeth developed a little cough. At first, this was not very noticeable, and sometimes, we didn't hear it for days. Within two weeks, however, it had become worse. The CPN had advised being very wary about such things, so I arranged a home visit from the doctor. Taking her to the local surgery would have been very difficult and hard work – she would not sit still at all. The Nurse Practitioner came out to see us, a really nice lady, who actually succeeded in taking Elspeth's temperature (in the ear), blood pressure and one or two other tests. I thought Elspeth wouldn't let her do this and would wriggle out of it all, but the nurse had a high degree of success! Antibiotics were prescribed. There was a mention of a chest X-ray, which concerned me, as I hadn't got a clue how we would keep Elspeth anywhere near an X-ray machine. I had visions of her having to be sedated but still wandering off, as she would not understand what was going on. We decided to give the antibiotics a chance and wait to see what would happen. For a week, the daytime wasn't too bad, but nights were pretty rough. As soon as she lay down, she started coughing. Nothing seemed to help with this, so we just had to put up with it for a pretty sleepless week. After that, there was still no improvement in her condition. The nurse rang to check on her progress, which I appreciated, and she arranged for a doctor to call on the same day. The doctor from the local surgery centre was brilliant, and she gave Elspeth a thorough check-over before prescribing a new dose of tablets, which was stronger this time. She asked all sorts of questions about the illness, taking lots of notes. I felt she was really trying to understand the whole situation. I was hoping to see an improvement in the near future. The cough cleared after what seemed like an eternity!

Meanwhile, my mum, at the age of ninety-four, began to have falls. She lived near Morecambe (where I was born). Being in Sheffield and with Elspeth so ill, I couldn't go over to see her as often as I wanted. My sister, who lived next door to her, had to deal with it all, which she did very well. The situation soon became more serious, and the decision was made to put 'Eileen' in a home near Carnforth. I received regular reports from my sister. After a while I learnt that Mum couldn't recognise any family from photos. She would ask, *'Who is that? What is his/her name?'* It seemed that in her old age, dementia had finally caught up with her. After hearing this news, it crossed my mind that it was such a tragedy life had not granted Elspeth the opportunity to at least grow old gracefully! My mum died not long before her ninety-seventh birthday. Elspeth was looked after by carers at home on the day of the funeral.

Moving on now, the next section features extracts from my annual newsletters to family and friends. I tried to keep everyone informed, from relatives to life-long friends, by sending a Christmas newsletter every year so that they would all be aware of the latest situation regarding Elspeth. The first of these follows on from where we have just left off.

2014

Hello everyone,

Time for the annual report. I'm afraid that, yet again, there is not a lot of good news regarding Elspeth. Sadly, I can't foresee any time in the future when there will be. Seems a shame that it is always this way when I write to you at Christmas, usually a time for being happy.

Elspeth continues to be well looked after by the care groups. We have the same hours and the same teams as always. The NHS did ring me up and say that there might have to be a change of agencies, but I haven't heard from them for weeks so I assume that we will be sticking with the same ones. To start with new carers would mean them all having to learn how to cope with Elspeth's difficulties from scratch. Lots of new faces in the house. Mmmm! I think we will be staying with the current teams.

Carers continue to take Elspeth out as often as possible, even when the weather is not so good. She has developed a habit of not getting out of the car on her return home. Fortunately, I have been present at those times and have been able to 'persuade' her out. Similarly, she sometimes refuses to get out of the bath, which is a problem for carers. She must be enjoying herself too much! I have had to 'haul' her out unceremoniously, and even though I am quite a big person, it was not an easy task.

She continues to eat very well. All you need to do is put a plate of food in front of her, and it goes as long as someone sits with her. Otherwise, she tends to take a mouthful and then walk. We still have to be careful not to leave food out, or that goes as well. Similarly, when she paints or does jigsaws, we have to sit with her, or she gets up to wander. Usually from the back door to the front door, always trying the handles. Maybe she has ideas for making a bid for freedom! Recently, we have had the doctor here three times. She has had a very bad cough, and no matter what medicines they gave her, it did not clear up. The first doctor prescribed antibiotics, which did not work at all after the course. The second was a lovely doctor from the local surgery, who prescribed stronger antibiotics and was very interested and caring with Elspeth. A week of those tablets didn't work either. The third doctor had seen Elspeth earlier in the year when she had three weeks of dizzy spells. He prescribed a nasal spray and if that didn't work in a week, some very strong antibiotics. The nasal spray did not work. It was more trouble than it was worth trying to push it up Elspeth's nose! She did not like it. So, we went on to the stronger antibiotics. Surprise, surprise! They didn't work either. Anyway, the cough seems slightly better now, so we'll just have to wait until it goes if it ever does. It is worrying because the immune system deteriorates as this illness worsens. She has also coughed lots in the middle of the night for several weeks now, which wakes me up. I'm not the world's best sleeper, and often, if I wake up at two or three in the morning, that is the end of my night. One or two short snoozes during the day have helped. I have a cough now!

Interestingly, Elspeth is sitting in my armchair in the front room and playing with Zoo, one of Alice's favourite cuddly toys, who lives downstairs at the moment. This is great when I come home, sometimes at five o'clock, because it means I can get on and prepare tea and I know exactly where she is. She will also sit and watch some television for a little while in the same chair. I used to put the Disney Channel on for her because I thought she liked the bright colours and movement, but I don't think it matters what's on!

Financially, we are coming to the end of her ISA (over £30,000), and we're soon going to have to dip into other savings. Elspeth will be getting her state pension soon, which will bring in another £111 a week. It will help, but it will all go on care fees. She hasn't got a lot saved elsewhere – except there is her part of the bond we took out years ago. When that goes, we may have to win the Lottery! The problem is we don't do it! Maybe there will be some extra Council help when she reaches the savings threshold of £23,500.

Three weeks ago, I went to look at a care home for possible respite care. It was in Gleadless, where I used to teach. The lady who showed me around had three daughters at my school some years earlier, and I had taught them all. It was a lovely place, and the staff were brilliant, but I decided against it in the end. It wasn't the cost because all we had to pay was £154 per week. Here at home, Elspeth has one-to-one care from 9.00 am to 5, 6 or 7.00 pm. The home I visited could not possibly offer that. They just do not have enough staff unfortunately. Also, Elspeth likes her daily rides and walks. The home could not offer that either. I had visions of her wandering up and down a lot. One suggestion is that our carers go into the home and look after her during the day. That could possibly be arranged with the agencies and the establishment itself. Maybe next year. A home will probably have to happen one day. There has been a big difference in Elspeth over the past twelve months. I think there will be an even bigger difference in the next year.

I am sure I will be writing another newsletter in a year's time, but I simply don't know what news will be in it. Nevertheless, I hope you all have a lovely Christmas and the best of New Years. We shall do our best to try!

2015

(The first of two this year)

Hello, all you peeps out there! Elspeth and I are fast approaching our thirty-ninth wedding anniversary – sixty-six and sixty-three years old, respectively also! How the years fly by. Happy birthday to us! Well, it's Christmas soon as well.

As this illness progresses, Elspeth needs to be guided a lot more and reminded of what to do in everyday situations. She regularly has to be pointed in the right direction to go somewhere, and she has to be shown how to carry out ordinary activities. When it clicks, she just gets on with it. Lately, she has been refusing to open her mouth to do her teeth in the morning, pushing the toothbrush away, etc. I have taken to giving her a towel to dry her hands on and putting the brush into her mouth when I can. Anyway, today is Tuesday and bath morning, so it's all someone else's job! She is finishing her breakfast off quietly with a carer at present.

There is not a lot of difference in her behaviour lately, just increasing vagueness. The consultant has reduced (quartered) her morning and evening quetiapine tablets down to the bare minimum, with a view to cutting them out altogether. This is what is done as Pick's advances. When the quetiapine stops, she will only be taking zopiclone sleeping tablets. I found out just how useful they were a week ago when, in a hurry, I thought I had given her zopiclone (not quetiapine) for her early evening tablet. I was advised not to give her any more tablets. She hardly slept a wink all night. She started leaning over me, pulling the duvet off or on – trying to be helpful. Or she found something to pick on my arm. It is not something I want at three in the morning, even though the dawn chorus is pleasant to listen to!

Now that the so-called warmer weather is here, Elspeth has begun, once again, to walk outside in the garden. She goes along the path to the garage and round to the carefully positioned (and locked) gate at the end of the passage. She can do this for a long time, back and forth, even though she uses the opportunity for a toilet break when on the move. Good thing there is a pants delivery this very day - I think we might need four pairs a day soon. Funnily enough, she will go into the garage loo, but she just stands there, not knowing what to do unless someone guides her. She often comes out having done nothing. She is eating well and healthily and still walks a lot on trips with the carers. Perhaps the reduction in her tablets will help her shed some of the weight she has put on over the past five years. The CPN says that the quetiapine may have contributed to her weight gain, which was considerable. Ah – I hear the bath running. Upstairs she goes, with a few of those by now customary short laughs. You always know where she is nowadays.

The carer will bathe Elspeth and wash her hair, then take her out for an hour or so. Normally, in term time, I will go up to school for choir practice, but of course it is now the great summer holidays. Instead, I will go to the supermarket and get the ingredients for a three-day bolognese, which saves cooking for two days. Also, Tuesday is a no pub, no booze day, so I need to find something to do. Test match tomorrow!

Last Monday, Elspeth came home with three bites on the back of her right hand. It became very swollen, and this lasted for five days. I think the Anthisan helped but you couldn't see the veins as it was so puffy. Seems ok but it was difficult trying to stop her scratching all the time. She was always a target for hungry horse flies. Another thing I am concerned about is that she needs a tooth taken out in September. That will be a fun time (not) as it involves injections, and as she is not keen on opening her mouth, I think we could have a stalemate. I need to talk again to the CPN but I do not relish the thought of the experience. Anyway, we persevere, although I have to say I look forward to the sessions when carers take her out, and I can have a little peace and quiet or get on with some jobs.

Annual barbecue on August the 8th to celebrate mine and Elspeth's birthdays and wedding anniversary. So sad she will not be a part of it after all these years but that's the way the cookie crumbles. I'll be in touch.

2015

I can't believe we are around to the Christmas newsletter again! The year has gone so quickly. Elspeth changes slowly but surely as her illness continues its relentless course. She now says nothing apart from the word 'yes.' Gone is any chance of conversation – it's been years since she said anything coherent. She has to be guided a lot more. She will still wash if she is passed the flannel, and do her teeth if prompted and helped. She has to be taken to the toilet and physically sat down. Sometimes she doesn't even realise she is still wearing her pants. We cannot have a fourth pair of pants per day; no one can, so I buy an extra pack or so each month. Hope it doesn't come to more than that as it's an expensive necessity. I am very grateful for the three pairs we do get, though the NHS may be cutting down in that area.

As some of you may know, Elspeth has had two hospital visits recently. The first was after a fall in the bedroom when she hurt her face. I was downstairs at the time, and she had gone to bed. She must have got up as I heard a loud bang on the ceiling. We took her to A&E, where she refused to be X-rayed – she wouldn't sit still long enough. She was badly bruised around her nose and eye, where she had hit the radiator, but the doctor reckoned there was nothing broken, so we went home after four hours. She did heal slowly. I now only give her the evening sleeping tablet when I go to bed, in case it was the zopiclone that made her very sleepy – enough to 'dozily' fall over. I don't know.

The second hospital visit was odd and almost a complete waste of an evening. The care agency rang me at 4.40 pm one day to say she was chewing something and would not spit it out. I went home, but none of us knew what it was, so I spent the next two hours trying to encourage her to spit it out. No luck here. In the end, I was concerned that she might get the object stuck in her throat when eating or sleeping, so I took her to A&E to see if they had any ideas. She was still sucking whatever it was (it felt hard like a small pebble). At 11 pm, she was falling asleep, so I told them we were going home. We'd have to chance it. Miraculously, we were told it was now our turn. Although the staff tried, no one had any real ideas, and she would not open her mouth, so we went home anyway. I tried coaxing her to open up, but suddenly, the object had gone! She had probably swallowed it with no after-effects. I hope we don't have another hospital trip for a long time. Talk about stubbornness! Would she open her mouth? Not on your life!

It has to be said that Elspeth has been quite a bit easier to deal with during the daytime. The Consultant has reduced her quetiapine dosage, and she now takes only one small tablet before tea. When she started this, the dose was eight times what it is now. There is a big risk of strokes with this tablet, so the medical people were keen to reduce her intake after all these years. She still takes the sleeping tablets late at night. If she doesn't, she has a bad night. There's less activity in the evening after she has gone to bed. Over the years, she has wandered to the toilet and back many times, but nowadays, she hardly makes one visit. As usual, when she goes there, she will probably come straight out and go back to bed. When I go to bed she is always awake and begins her ritual of scratching my arm and adjusting the duvet. She will lean over me for a long time. I leave the radio on Classic FM all evening for her to listen to. Looming over me in the light cast by the radio, she looks quite eerie in the early hours of the morning.

The mental health staff and I have been once again talking about the possibility of a home. I don't want to do this yet, as Elspeth is not ready. I believe she knows her way around the house, and she gives the impression that she is happy here. It would be good if we knew what she actually felt, as it is all guesswork with her. She still spends a lot of time wandering between the front door and the back door. They are locked, and she still tries to go out through the door and down the road. In the past she has 'escaped' but not walked very far before one of us has caught up with her. Careless on our part, but it's so difficult to be always watching her. She continues to enjoy colouring, simple painting, and, at times, jigsaws, but she has to have a carer with her so she doesn't immediately stand up and walk about. Her appetite is still excellent, but you need to play a game with her when it comes to meals, as she forgets how to eat. You give her a spoonful, and then she takes a spoonful, and so on.

Recently we had what could have been bad news over funding from Social Services. They wanted to take away her travel allowance, which is over £3000 p/a. Their contribution is part of a split package with the NHS, which began with them putting over £600 per month towards this package. That went down over the years to £467. If they took away the mileage allowance, it would reduce their contribution to less than £200 per month. I felt I needed to discuss this, so I e-mailed to explain how trips out were one of the few things that gave Elspeth pleasure nowadays. To cut a long story short, the allowance was reinstated, and I received a long e-mail explaining why, all to do with Elspeth's well-being. I was very relieved not to lose this money because life is very expensive at present. We have to find a lot of money every month to keep this vital package going. I think the overall cost is around £45,000 p/a, and our contribution is sizeable.

The NHS contacted me to say it was time for Elspeth's review. She hadn't had one for a long time. A representative came, and we went through all the information we had about Elspeth and her various needs. I got the impression that I was going to be told she didn't require nursing, which is true at the moment. Then, I suddenly thought that her funding was going to be reduced. The man saw Elspeth for a while, as I had purposely asked her carer not to take her out, and then, to my intense relief, he firmly said that the package would stay the same. It had to go to the panel, but I am sure the NHS will continue to fund their twenty-two hours a week, plus mileage. Budgets should include money for those like Elspeth, who is very seriously mentally ill. I still don't think many people understand the extra challenges of Pick's disease. You need to go to the many websites and read the information. This illness may last twelve years or more but often terminates at seven or eight. The body's immune system weakens and then may stop working properly, so other illnesses, such as pneumonia, will be fatal. Elspeth is already seven or eight years into that time. Happy days. Again, I have no idea what my news will be like in a year's time, but we will deal with that when it comes. I hope you all enjoy yourselves and have a brilliant Christmas. Maybe a few glasses of wine, etc.

2016

Hello all!

A year has passed, and it is again time to write my annual newsletter to keep you all up to date with events in the Faraday family. It has not been the greatest year, but we have survived. Elspeth is now off pills, apart from her sleeping tablet, and there has been little noticeable difference in her behaviour. She has lost a lot of weight – up to three stones so far, which has been put down to not taking any quetiapine. She looks better, and I am even thinking of trying to resurrect some of her earlier clothing, which might now fit her. She is still walking a lot at home and out with her carers. This has always been and still is her favourite activity. Everybody says that she is slower than she used to be and she doesn't like going up hills. Lately, she has adopted a more 'plodding' style of walking. As I write now, at this moment, she is walking between the front door and the kitchen door clutching a school-type paintbrush! We have had to block off the staircase because if she saw a way up, she would think it was bedtime and go up to put her nightie on at any time in the day.

Sadly, she has now completely lost the power of speech and has not said a word for a few months. This is part of the progress of Pick's disease. Our house is now very quiet for most of the time, which is most unusual for our family. Carers and I speak to her as normal, but not a lot will go in. She certainly doesn't understand what anyone says, and she does not seem to recognise anyone. Well, maybe she still knows me, as I see her more than anybody else. I don't know for certain.

Nighttimes are again becoming more and more frustrating. Elspeth goes to bed, as usual, after 7.30 pm, and we might not hear anything for a while. Then, there will be footsteps on the ceiling, and she will walk around on the landing. She likes to go to the top of the stairs, look down the stairs, and then go back to the bedroom. I am not sure whether it frightens her to come downstairs by herself but she still does that on the odd occasion. I wonder whether it is when she doesn't feel well, but as she can't tell us, we don't know, or we have to guess what's wrong. When I go to bed, she is awake, and then the poking and scratching begins!

The Occupational Therapist (OT) came around a little while ago and suggested we had a second handrail installed on the stairs, for extra safety. This would give Elspeth confidence. The lady said she could arrange for the fitting, but we would have to pay for the rail itself. I haven't heard anything about this recently, but I hope it will materialise in the near future. It will cost about £40, which is good value.

I am a bit concerned about the continence situation, as the NHS may not be able to find the same finance for this department. There is talk of a 'pant reduction'! We'll have to wait and see. Three pairs a day is our allocation, and I buy enough for a fourth if needed. If I had to buy all of them, it would probably cost well in excess of £1000 p/a. The thought of another extra cost was very concerning. Apparently, the NHS department has a new supplier, and the carers say the quality of the new pants is not as good. Looks like the washing machine might be in use a lot more next year since even the good quality pants she has at the moment do not completely stop the occasional wetting of beds and clothing. One piece of advice – check there aren't any continence pads in the washing machine amongst other articles of clothing etc. The pads disintegrate and cover everything else with fluff, which is a total pain to clean off!

After Christmas, Elspeth is going to be discharged from the mental health team's books. Our CPN has been with us since the start of all this, many years ago, and she has been magnificent. I have much to thank her for. The reason for the discharge is that Elspeth has reached a stage in her illness where they cannot do much more for her. In fact, when the CPN comes to see me once a month, there is not an awful lot of change in Elspeth's condition to discuss. If I need to, I can contact the team in the future. I think the visits are due to stop in February or March next year. The plan is to pass Elspeth's care on to our local surgery and put her under the care of the GPs there. If so, they'll have to understand the situation and not ring me up asking to speak to her!

Elspeth has begun to be fed more at meal times. She does lose interest and we have to fill her spoon and put it into her mouth. She tends to sip at a drink, so it takes a long time for her to have a cold drink or a coffee. We are told she needs at least eight drinks a day, but it's a difficult target to meet and takes a lot of time and patience.

I am still being asked whether I would like some respite care. My answer is yet again that Elspeth seems happy at home; maybe she even knows where she is. If she was put in a home for a week the cover would not be the same as she has here, and I have a picture in my mind of her walking around lost. The staff are brilliant in the homes I have visited, but there are simply not enough to give her equivalent care to the one-to-one care she receives at our home.

Funding from the NHS was agreed for the next three years or so. Thank goodness! Who knows what condition Elspeth will be in by then? This is a pretty disheartening stage of our lives, but the most important thing is to keep her happy, whatever that means. Our fortieth wedding anniversary was on August 5th this year. We had a nice barbecue on the Saturday nearest to that date and I invited the usual group of lovely, old friends. Elspeth had no idea what was going on, even though some of them went in to see her. A carer looked after her and put her to bed. I wasn't even able to take her out for a celebration meal, as I used to do in the old days.

I hope your Christmas is happy and peaceful. We shall certainly do our best to make it that way here in Sheffield!

2017

Well, here I am sitting next to Elspeth on Sunday, the 4th of November. As usual, I am administering her evening meal, which takes an hour and a half on average, spoonful by slow spoonful. She actually loves it, but it is certainly a major event. She will feed herself puddings – she obviously has a sweet tooth. After she has eaten she will go to bed. Then, surprisingly, as long as she is well, there will be no more bother until the morning. I sometimes find her in the same position as the one she adopted when she went to bed. Give her a teddy bear and some gentle music and she is sorted. How different from a year or two ago, when she was wandering about turning taps on or finding all manner of odd things to do. She has to be washed, dressed, and mostly fed. Due to difficulties putting her in the bath I had the bathroom converted into a wet room with a shower only. This is proving to be a hit with the carers, as showering makes everyone's life just that bit easier. I also spent some of her DLA on a shower chair that can be adjusted up and down with a remote control. The plumber did a fine job, but the new room also suits me!

When out for a walk now, carers must link arms or hold hands. Elspeth is not as steady on her feet as she used to be, but she still enjoys going out for car rides and walks if there are not many people about. I think crowds are bothering her.

This is a busy month for a lot of reasons. Elspeth had a flu injection on Friday, which should have been at our house, but the local surgery said that she is not eligible for a home visit anymore. This is after seven years of home visits. After the injection, there is a dementia review, then a gynecological review at the hospital, followed by one or two other visits from people, including the dentist—all necessary stuff. Alzheimer's Society is stopping its Outreach work at the end of March next year, as their budget is not being renewed, so we lose Thursday and Friday mornings. There will be others who will lose out far more. We will just have to find ways around it that don't cost more money. Of course this means I will be further tied to the house on those mornings, but that's the way it goes.

I don't have a clue about how many more years this illness will continue since it is already twelve years since it (probably) started. At times, I sit and think what a waste it has been of what should have been the best years.

I hope Elspeth is well over the next couple of weeks as I have a very important Christmas concert to do and besides that Alice's group is putting on an anniversary concert to mark twenty years of their existence, even though they don't sing together regularly anymore. That should be a lot of fun. I have cover until 11.30 pm that night. Free of charge, as it's a friend.

It is now almost December and I can report that all the appointments went well. In particular, the gynaecologist and nurse were superb, as was the dentist. We are so lucky to have such good service. We don't need to go back for four and six months, respectively.

Today, I received a letter discharging Elspeth from the mental health team's books. Ten years they have been with her, and they know her better than anyone else. What a shame they are finishing. The CPN has advised and guided us through some tricky times and never let us down. I know she can't do much more for Elspeth, but I feel rather apprehensive about not having her here for advice and help. We will soldier on. If the agencies raise their charges I will have to cut more hours. We are reaching a difficult stage, I fear.

Have a great Christmas and lots of jollity. I would love El to take part, as she used to, but for obvious reasons she can't.

2018

Well, where do I begin? So much has happened in the last year. There is a big difference in Elspeth, particularly over the last six months. She is not sleeping very well at night again, probably because she goes to sleep a lot during the day when she is sitting in a chair or in the back seat of a carer's car. I often find her in the middle of the night playing with a teddy bear or two when she should be asleep. She recently went through a habit of sliding out of bed and sitting on the floor in the early hours. It took a great deal of effort to put her back into bed, as it was like lifting a large sack of potatoes! A dead weight. I hope my back can stand it all, or we could be in trouble. That seems to have stopped now, for the time being and nights are a bit better. Lately she has had two or three falls, which have been to do with slippery ground and not failing limbs. The latest one, although she was with a carer, was by our front gate before the pavement had been resurfaced. Sheffield has been re-doing the surfaces of roads and pavements for a while now, and ours were due. She gave herself two black eyes and bruised knees. Two days later, she had a really bad night and was making strange noises all night. No sleep for anyone. The following day, we were all worried about her breathing, and an ambulance was called. The first responder put an oxygen mask on her, and the ambulance took her up to the hospital to be checked out. Some hours later, I was told she had a chest infection, and she was put on antibiotics. They had difficulty, of course, in diagnosing what was wrong with her as she could not tell them anything. This causes major problems, as you can imagine but I was very pleased with what they did for her. It seems to have cleared up now, but we need to return to attempt a second X-ray before Christmas to check everything is ok.

Elspeth has had some bleeding lately and was found to have a prolapse, which is just our luck to add to everything else. More hospital visits and another reason for everybody to be careful on walks and in general. She has again developed a bad habit of putting things in her mouth. We have had problems with this as she won't open her mouth to let us take things out. The latest was an olive stone, mistakenly given her at lunch, which we 'flipped out' using a toothbrush. Next, she succeeded in eating a small rubber from the end of a pencil. She had swallowed it before I could do much. I assume that by now it has passed safely through! She has taken to watching television more, and when I make tea I just sit her down in a comfortable chair and put the TV on. This is very useful as I know where she is, and she enjoys playing with a teddy bear at the same time. We have also had a funding review from the NHS and Social Services, and we are keeping the same funding. This is some good news due to the huge cost of her care package. I can't think what life would be like if we didn't have that care package. Carers are continuing to have car problems with Elspeth, as she often refuses to get in or out for some reason. You will remember that she loves to go out for walks and drives, so we are baffled by this. She spent forty-five minutes once when I was not present, refusing to come out of the back of one carer's car.

We have no idea what we shall be doing at Christmas this year, but there is no doubt that it will be very merry. We shall have to play it by ear due to the fact that Catriona had a baby girl this month, born at 2lb 12 oz. She (Anya) is coming along fine and putting on weight, which is great news. It is so sad that Elspeth will never know Anya properly, but we will introduce her to her granny as often as possible.

2019

Well, I need to make a start sometime, although this one is going to be quite difficult. In this last year there has been the biggest deterioration yet in Elspeth's condition. She is tired all the time now and falls asleep, even at breakfast. Carers are very good with her and sit patiently waiting for her to wake up. She spends thirteen or fourteen hours a day in bed, but I am not sure how much she sleeps or whether the sleeping tablet is now having any effect. I begin to wonder whether it's worth stopping the zopiclone. She has had her flu injection and, so far this year, has stayed relatively free from illness – touch wood! We are still having to guess if there is a problem because, as you know, she hasn't used coherent speech for the last two years, ever since the illness affected that part of her brain.

Her incontinence has been more under control in the last months, particularly since the hospital changed the pessary she has to wear due to her prolapse. Thank goodness for that. To put it bluntly, we have had some pretty messy experiences. She is becoming more fussy about eating and, in particular drinking lately. We have to spend a long time to get even the minimum amount of liquid or food down her, as she is very good at refusing to open her mouth. She 'pouches' food in her cheeks, and it all has to be scooped out – not the most pleasant activity – so it is important we get into her mouth. Difficult! We saw the dentist yesterday for a check-up and mentioned this. She suggested a visit from the speech therapist, who may be able to advise us on swallowing techniques. We'll see if it does any good.

Elspeth has developed a dangerous habit of leaning backwards when she is standing, which we have got to watch. She is also more and more unsteady on her feet. She cannot walk as far as she used to, and someone has to be close to her to make sure she doesn't fall over. This began a few weeks ago when I brought her downstairs in the morning. As usual, she went into the front room to stand and stare out of the window. I heard a loud bang and found her sitting on the floor next to the fireplace. She was okay but it certainly means we can't let her out of our sight again. I stand close behind her when dressing her or brushing her hair in front of the hall mirror, as she tends to lean back on me. Besides the new handrail I had put on the stairs, I have also put up a lot of grab rails for her to hold on to, as she can still climb slowly up the stairs (with someone behind her), and this helps tremendously.

It could be that we are due for a stairlift in the next twelve months or so. Once she is upstairs, she is once again going to bed and staying there with her favourite teddy bear. Evenings are a little more relaxing downstairs.

Catriona and her family have recently moved to a bigger house, and we are all invited there for Christmas Day, which means we shall take Elspeth – and stay in a different house! That will be interesting – they have a steep staircase. We'll see how it goes! I am applying for PIP payments instead of DLA, ever hopeful that I'll receive a bit more money to help with the care bills. The form took a week to fill in! I'm hoping to hear from the DWP soon.

That's about it for this Christmas. Time to print out and start the Christmas cards. Have a great time, everybody – we will do our best!

2020

An interesting year, to say the least. Sorry to say that the deterioration in Elspeth's health continues, slowly but surely. We continue to help her everywhere, as this habit of leaning backwards is giving us great cause for concern. Someone must support her. Stairs are a big problem for the agency carers, with some, because of the possible dangers, not wanting to take her up or downstairs anymore, which means I must do it. I don't find it difficult but great care is needed. She clutches onto the bannisters and has a very strong grip. I have to prise her hands off to be able to go up or down. There is still talk of a stairlift, but not yet. We recently did get an NHS toilet seat (I thought you'd like to know!), one of those with handles that you can lift, and that seems to be a hit. Cold, though, at this time of year, in the garage loo! She sits most of the time during the day and can only walk very short distances accompanied by a carer, but she goes out most days, generally for a ride. Due to all the sitting and time spent in bed, she has to have a variety of creams and sprays administered so as to avoid skin complaints. She still goes to bed at the usual time, which gives me a free evening, and she will stay in bed the following day till various times, depending on who is coming to us.

Lately Elspeth has been making a series of loud, bizarre noises during the night, which doesn't help anyone's sleep, but there is not a lot we can do about that. I cannot sleep in another room in case anything happens, although that is now unlikely, as she has remained quite still in bed for some years now. I still give her a sleeping pill at night, but I am not convinced that it now does anything for her. I can hear her snoring but I'm unsure as to how much sleep she gets. Her cognition is virtually non-existent, but you can still see a skill in the way she handles a paintbrush, although she is only painting water onto an invisible picture. She likes watching others colouring in her books. No small objects are used or left out because she has a habit of putting them into her mouth, and that, as we have already found out, leads to problems and a possible hospital trip. We are very careful. The team of carers is excellent and does everything for her. Some of them have been with Elspeth for years and know her very well. They really enjoy coming to look after her. That might be because she is one of their younger clients, at sixty-eight years old. Her appetite is brilliant, and she will just keep on eating if we provide her with food. She has a great menu, mostly home-cooked food – including fresh fruit, vegetables, yoghurts, etc. I spend quite a lot of time preparing and cooking interesting dishes for her. Tonight, she's having rice pudding with chocolate cake. Well, you can't be healthy all the time! Her weight is good, and she doesn't seem to be putting any on, even though she doesn't exercise much anymore. So, we are looking after her well, bearing in mind that this illness should last between two and twelve years, and she's beyond that already. The pandemic hasn't made any difference to her life because she is in her own little world. As long as she can eat, sleep, join in an activity or two, and be taken out, nothing else really matters. She has not been aware of the lockdown. We both had flu jabs and the Covid jab is next on the list—full marks to the carers, who have not missed a day during this period so far. I have managed to redecorate most of the house and we've had a lot of roof work done – and a new gas boiler soon. I haven't been sitting down and doing nothing!

Catriona is due to have another baby on December 20th, although the families are running a sweepstakes on the date. She knows it will be a boy who will be called Robin. I note that Sheffield is to remain in tier three after lockdown, which means that as Elspeth has regular carers, I can go to visit Cat and family in a bubble whenever I want.

Although the news of Elspeth is not good, we shall all do our best for her over the Christmas period to try and give her as happy a time as possible. She will be totally unaware of what's going on, but I hope that she will feel relaxed and happy within herself. She will certainly get plenty of one of her favourite activities, which is eating!

It just remains for me to wish you all a very happy Christmas and New Year. I hope you have a brilliant time. I will be in touch next year.

2021

It's only the middle of November, but I will make a start on this year's news. It has been a busy year. Elspeth's mobility is very poor, and walking any distance is out of the question. She moves with difficulty, supported by carers or myself. She has fallen a few times, but as she has support, she has not hurt herself. The most she can do is a short tour of the downstairs of our house, guided by two of us. We have managed to take her into the garden, down to the summer house once a week, so she can have a change of scenery and sit out. I think she enjoys this 'activity'.

Elspeth now sleeps downstairs in the dining room, which has been converted into a bedroom for her. We have a hospital bed in there. The stairlift idea has been dropped. I had to clear a lot of furniture and other bits and pieces, but this change is working very well. It was both sad and strange at first not to have her in our bedroom after forty-five years. But now I have a bed to myself upstairs, and when she makes those odd noises during the night, I can hardly hear her, so I actually get more sleep. She sleeps quite a bit during the day, especially when she is in front of the television in the special chair with her legs up. The District Nurse said she should do this for at least an hour a day, as it helps when her ankles swell up due to lack of exercise. She also seems to get a lot of blisters for some inexplicable reason—great, big ones on her fingers and toes. Doctors didn't seem too concerned, and the blisters do go away after a few days.

Carers have been told that due to health and safety, they should no longer help me take her upstairs for a shower, so I have to do that by myself, which is becoming increasingly more difficult and dangerous.

They still do the shower, after I have taken her upstairs. Going up is a slow job, as she has trouble raising her left foot to reach the next step. It won't be too long before I won't be able to do this, and she will have to have a bed or chair wash downstairs, which is not as thorough. I have bought a hair bath to solve the hair washing problem. So, she spends most of her time in the old dining room, looking at books and videos with the carers whilst clutching a couple of teddy bears. She was always fascinated by teddy bears. Remember when she made about a hundred and twenty named badges for the nurses at the Children's Hospital? She was most concerned when one turned up at a car boot sale we had gone to!

One carer still takes her down to sit in the summer house. This is a major operation and involves two of us. It is very slow, but it gives her a change of surroundings and I am sure she enjoys it. They listen to podcasts and folk music. Sometimes, he plays the guitar and sings.

One great thing happened recently, which was an enormous relief. There was a big drop in monthly payments to Sheffield Council. After fifteen years of expenditure on care fees, Elspeth's savings had dropped below the £23,500 threshold, and her contributions were reduced from £424 per week to £52! Maybe we will recuperate a small amount of the six figures we have spent over the years. Because of this, life is a bit easier financially at present.

We have both had our flu and three Covid jabs and fortunately stayed clear of illness, probably mostly because Elspeth does not meet crowds of people. She did have a virus a few weeks ago, which gave her a nasty cough for four weeks and antibiotics took a while to work. It's gone now, thank goodness.

We still visit the hospital for her gynaecological needs. It's the four-monthly visit soon. That's a job in itself as we have to have wheelchairs and hoists organised. Still, after that, we should have a pretty clear run-up to Christmas. Normally, we would go up to Catriona's for the meal, but we are not able to move Elspeth too much now. So, Alice and her partner Richie are coming to me for the Christmas Eve and Christmas Day meal. The rest of the family will join us in the evening for some hilarity. They will stay the night, so there should be a full house. I hope we're not too noisy as Elspeth will be next to us in the dining room. How she would have loved to join in with Christmas. For the first time I have had to book carers on Christmas day, as I need extra expert help with getting Elspeth up in the morning and putting her to bed.

Oh, by the way, Robin was born a couple of weeks late, on January the 1st. His arrival came just after last year's newsletter. Like his sister Anya, we will introduce him to Granny as often as possible. Sadly, she will never hold him and will never realise who he is. But at least she will have met both her grandchildren.

Best wishes for a very happy Christmas and a marvellous New Year.

2022

Here we go again! I hope you are all well and escaping Covid and other illnesses. Elspeth and I have had our Covid boosters and flu injections, so I hope we're covered. Her deterioration is to be expected. I think it's over fifteen years since her initial MRI and brain scans. She had to give up walking last year and we have had a ceiling hoist installed in her bedroom, the former dining room, which was kindly paid for by Sheffield Council. Carers have been receiving hoist training. The Council is also putting more money in, which pays for much of her sixty hours plus of care per week. This is, of course, since she reached the savings threshold. I am very grateful for this help. Elspeth hardly leaves her room. She has all her meals in there and sits for the day. We try to find activities for her but they are limited. We need to keep some form of stimulation going on in her head.

Two carers come in the morning and evening to get her up and put her to bed. They use the hoist to place her in a chair after doing the personal care that I used to do, which is good news for me. I give her breakfast and make some lunches and all her evening meals. During the week, we probably have a dozen or more carers who visit, and also two District Nurses who come to check on bed sores, etc. It is quite busy here. We now take her into the front room using a wheelchair lent to us by the NHS. We had to do this when the piano tuner came recently, as our piano was in Elspeth's bedroom, and he needed the room to himself! I purchased some ramps, so we also managed to wheel her outside and down to sit under the old apple tree at the bottom of the garden for lunch when the weather was warmer. She is still making a lot of bizarre noises and sleeping for most of the day or eating for the rest of it. What has happened to her over the past twenty years is a tragedy. No one really knows the causes of Pick's disease. Maybe one day, when it's too late for us, there will be a huge discovery! I am eternally grateful for the excellent care she receives.

I think the most difficult part of the situation is the fact that Elspeth cannot talk to us and tell us, in particular, what is the matter with her if we think she's not feeling well. Instead of speaking, she tends to make her noises for most of the day and night, and we are never sure what these mean, or whether she is trying to tell us something. She has begun coughing loudly when eating or drinking and has been prescribed a drinks thickener to combat this. Some of her noises will be due to the illness, but not being able to talk and explain makes life difficult for her and everyone.

So that's it for another year. As usual, I am not sure what the next twelve months will bring, but I haven't been sure for years. No difference there.

I hope you all have a very happy Christmas and an excellent New Year.

Cheers, and love to all.

2023

It's been quite a year! As many of you know, Elspeth had two sessions in hospital, the first of which was very serious, involving pneumonia and sepsis. We took her in by ambulance (fabulous paramedics, as always), and the doctor was quick to tell us the problem. She was given a 50/50 chance of surviving. I sat with her as long as I could, till the early hours. She seemed to be holding on, so I went home, expecting to be back later that morning. I didn't sleep as I was waiting for the phone to ring at any moment. It did at about 4.00 am, but it was the wrong number. Panic over for the time being. I visited Elspeth every day for four weeks. She was on oxygen from a mask and strong antibiotics through a drip. It took the whole month, but she never gave up and came through it, making an unexpected recovery. She was declared medically fit and brought home by ambulance after twenty-eight days. What a fighter! 'Non Deficere'! We had to deal with the catheter she had, which was removed after a couple of weeks. That made life a bit easier for everyone.

Not many weeks after this, she was back in hospital, but this time with a virus. Once again, we went in by ambulance at midnight, and I arrived home at 8.00 am. Back to the usual car-parking chaos at the hospital later that day! But this time, there was no oxygen or antibiotics needed, and to my relief, she was back home in four days.

Since the second hospital stay, Elspeth has been in bed at home. This has been for many weeks, but recently the NHS provided us an adjustable chair for her to sit in. It's on casters so that we can take her into another room for a change of environment. We had a visit from the Occupational Therapist to check the chair and fit a new electric cushion, which was an interesting procedure involving a pair of sharp scissors. We can put her in the chair for short sessions, building up to the maximum over the next few weeks.

One morning, the carers found a lump under one of Elspeth's breasts. That was all we needed. The doctor came and checked it out. We told him that Elspeth's mother had had breast cancer. He did not know whether it was cancer or not, and due to the Pick's, the best thing to do was nothing. He must have known something we didn't. Anyway, the lump did not appear to bother Elspeth again. She was soon used to the chair and began to enjoy it very much. We have to build her muscles up in order for her to sit properly, so she is hoisted in for half-hour sessions. Then, longer and longer until, hopefully, by Christmas, she will be able to sit all day. We position her by the patio window, looking out into the garden. It's really good to see her out of bed after the time she has spent lying there over the past few weeks. Apart from vocalising, she does very little nowadays. Carers try to involve her in activities, but there is not a lot that they, or she, can do. At least she eats well and has a good menu. All food now has to be puréed, so I have invested in an electric whisk and blending accessories. She also needs what is known as level 4 drinks thickener – seven scoops! This helps to prevent her from coughing and choking. Almost anything can be puréed, so she gets the flavours, but she has to miss the fun of being able to chew. She did have a great knowledge of food and inherited her mother's cooking skills, so I like to think that she appreciates the cauliflower cheese, hummus and avocado vinaigrette I give her. Also, lots of slow-cooked stews – which, when puréed, look a bit like cow pat – and also mashed potato with butter or horse radish and so on. Puréed brussels sprouts and carrots have an interesting appearance but taste fine.

More carers come and go to keep Elspeth clean and fresh. After they put her to bed in the evening, she invariably makes her noises for hours. I am in the front room, next to her, and I can still hear her, even when wearing my earphones. It becomes very wearing after a while. It is a relief when she goes to sleep, but often, that is not for too long. I feel lucky when it is quiet for a whole evening. I am very glad that she has her bed downstairs in the dining room, as I can get some degree of peace due to sleeping upstairs. We take each day as it comes.

And so, yet another Christmas and another newsletter. I would think we're closing in on twenty now. How things have changed further.

2024

(Written June 2024)

There will be no Christmas newsletter this year, as Elspeth passed away on the 26th of April. She had a good Christmas. Carers don't normally come on Christmas Day, but I booked some extra care in order to have time to make Christmas dinner for her, my daughter Alice, husband Richie, and Elspeth's brother Ruairidh, who also came with cousin Jo at New Year. Everything seemed to be going well.

Throughout January, it was clear that Elspeth was not one hundred per cent happy, but we managed to get through to February without any major mishaps. When February came, I was in touch with the doctors on a few occasions when she had high temperatures. She was put on a couple of courses of antibiotics, but these didn't seem to do much to help her.

Then, at the end of the month, the twenty-sixth to be precise, she was not at all well in the early evening. She had another high temperature and was sweaty and clammy. She seemed to be struggling to breathe, so I called an ambulance. The paramedics arrived and once again were marvellous. They put an oxygen mask on her to help with the breathing. The carers and I were standing out of the way, just watching and hoping, when Elspeth went into respiratory arrest. I remember seeing her face turn blue as the paramedics worked on her. They calmly dealt with the situation. It was a dreadful minute or so for everybody. I wasn't sure what was happening and thought that was it. I asked the paramedics whether she had 'gone.' Suddenly, Elspeth came around and began breathing again. The colour came back to her face. She had had a seizure. I went to the hospital with her in the ambulance with the lights flashing and the sirens going. It did not take long to arrive there.

Elspeth was seen by a Consultant, and the outlook seemed bleak. However, after seventeen days of oxygen, antibiotics, and hospital, she was back at home and discharged. I could not believe it, as I truly thought that her fight was over. But it wasn't! She was not ready to give up.

Elspeth had three or four weeks at home before she had to go back into hospital again on the eighth of April. I had no hesitation in calling for an ambulance, as the symptoms were the same as before. This time, the talk with the doctors was all about the end of life. I had already agreed on a DNR (do not resuscitate – a document stating that someone should not be resuscitated following cardiac arrest) for her, which I felt was an awful thing to have to do, but it was unnecessary in the end. When I walked out of the hospital building to go home there was a very eerie atmosphere in the ambulance parking area. No vehicles, no taxis, just unusually silent and still and dark.

Elspeth was once again given a bed in the geriatric ward amongst older ladies, and my endless visits began once more. By now, I had worked out that to claim a parking space in the hospital car park, it was wise to go later in the day, when day staff were going home, and there were more spaces. This was a much better plan and I had no problem for the remainder of my hospital visits.

I did feel I was being gently prepared for the end, as there was not a lot more that the hospital could do. Much of the conversation with doctors was about how to keep Elspeth comfortable. She was taken off oxygen and drip antibiotics (these, though strong, were not working), and she was not eating or drinking much at all. I remember seeing her legs once, which were so thin due to the muscles disappearing through inactivity.

After a few days, I was asked whether I wanted Elspeth to stay in the hospital or go into a nursing home. The other choice would have been to come home, which was out of the question since she was so ill. I was given the details of three or four nursing homes near where we lived, so I did some visiting and chose one. The NHS would fully fund the care. She was moved into the nursing home of my choice on Monday, the twenty-second of April. I made my daily visits, along with one or two of her carers, who wanted to see her. I was asked if I wanted a chaplain's visit. Also, a member of the staff at Saint Luke's Hospice, which supports and cares for people affected by terminal illness, came to talk with me.

On Thursday afternoon, I visited the home, and it was a strange visit, as I now recall. I talked with Elspeth as she lay in bed, staring into space, not seeming to notice me. I stayed about an hour before getting up to go home. The last thing I did was walk to the window to have a look at the garden area just outside. As I did this, I noticed her eyes were following me, and she was turning her head towards me. She had not done this for a long, long time. I leant over her and gave her a kiss, telling her I would be back the following day and I would stay longer. Her eyes followed me as I left the room.

I thought nothing more of this as I went home and spent a quiet evening before going to bed at about eleven o'clock. I was sleeping when the phone rang at about half past midnight. I missed the call because I was asleep, but a voicemail had been left, asking me to come into the nursing home and telling me Elspeth had stopped breathing. I went in and was taken to her room, where she was lying in bed, just as I had left her some hours before. The bed was neatly made, and the room was spotlessly tidy. Elspeth's mouth was slightly open, her eyes were closed, and her face had a yellowish tinge to it. She looked very peaceful, more at rest than I had seen for a long time. I sat with her and spoke to her, my hand on her shoulder. After nearly forty-eight years of married life, it was an incredibly poignant few minutes. I kissed her forehead, which was cold, said goodbye, and left the room. The staff saw me out. I was told the doctor was on his way to the nursing home to certify the death, and Elspeth's body would be moved out within the next few hours.

It was the saddest journey of my life, that short trip back home. Images of dozens of events flash through my mind. The one that kept coming back was Elspeth's face and eyes following me around her room. I will never forget that. It was as if she knew what was about to happen.

At home, I sat in my chair for a little while to pull my thoughts together and then made some phone calls to family, abruptly waking them up in the early hours. I went to bed at about three-thirty and did not sleep much. There was much to do later that day.

In Conclusion - 2024

(Written 21.06.24)

Later on that morning, there were a lot of phone calls to make to such places as the DWP (for pension and PIP), the solicitor, the bank, the funeral directors, and other establishments. I still had outstanding payments to make for the final care fees, but unfortunately, the bank had frozen the Deputy's bill-paying account, and I had to go in to close it and get them to transfer the money into my current account. Due to Elspeth's many days in hospital when there was no care to pay for, there was quite a large surplus sum (over £8,000) to return to the council, which they would naturally want back! Catriona and I called in at the bank, which happened to be opposite the town hall, so we collected the death certificate first. Well, we had to because the bank needed their own copy. I also made appointments to sort out the arrangements for Elspeth's funeral, which would be within the next fortnight.

It was a morning (sorry about the pun) funeral held at the crematorium near where we live. A lot of people came to say their goodbyes to Elspeth, including many cousins, other members of her large family, and some life-long friends. The celebrant was excellent and gave a wonderful presentation about Elspeth's life, which we had discussed a few days earlier. Everyone agreed that the service was very fitting and a lovely tribute to Elspeth. At the end, our family stood together quietly by the coffin for a moment before leaving the crematorium. The exit music was 'The Dashing White Sergeant,' a favourite folk tune, which Elspeth would have approved of and which brought a smile to everyone's face.

The wake and buffet were held at our local pub. People were more relaxed there and enjoyed 'catching up' with those they had not seen for years. Elspeth always loved folk music and ceilidh dancing, and she would have so enjoyed the music and clog-dancing (that's right – clog-dancing!) which took place later on in the afternoon. Perhaps she was watching and joining in!

Elspeth had told Alice many years before that she wanted her ashes to be scattered at Theddlethorpe, on the east coast. This was where she and her family had spent many happy hours picnicking and playing amongst the dunes. Catriona booked a holiday house in Lincolnshire for a weekend in June so we could carry out Elspeth's wishes. The 8th was a beautiful, sunny Saturday – a little breezy, though. The family and I walked a long way out towards the sea and said our final farewells before scattering the ashes, each in turn. We then went back towards the dunes for a nostalgic picnic.

So what now? After an incredibly challenging twenty years and more, the wheel has turned a full circle, and Elspeth is at peace. Although the whole experience was extremely demanding, I am proud of what we all achieved for her. What should have been the best part of our lives was taken away. There was no alternative but to make her life as comfortable and happy as possible under the circumstances. The course of Pick's disease is slow and persistent, and I often wonder, 'Why Elspeth?' but there is no answer to that. Why anybody? I think of other people who must be undergoing the same 'test,' and I sincerely hope they have the strength and courage to see it through. I think I survived by filling any spare time with activities to occupy my mind, such as my work with children and young people. If I had just become sad and depressed, that would have surely finished me off. There were some quiet moments where I would sit and think about things by myself, but I constantly told myself to never give up on Elspeth and to deal with every challenge as it arose – and there were many. I also wanted to do my best for my girls and all the friends who helped over the years. The knowledge that I had a beautiful family was a constant source of comfort during the worst times. I will not miss the worry and uncertainty that we all went through, not knowing what Elspeth's constant noises meant or whether she was in pain and couldn't tell us. Should I call the doctor? Should I call an ambulance? What should I do next to solve so many difficult problems? And then there was that feeling of apprehension, which sometimes would not go away. But my mind is clearer today, and I can breathe more easily, although there is now a missing link in my life.

Looking back the whole process involved so many difficulties. However, I think of the many carers who came to our house to look after Elspeth, all of them doing a brilliant job, all filled with cheerful, good humour and the desire to help her and improve her quality of life. I think of the wonderful service given to us by the doctors and nurses at the hospital, the ambulance service, the CPN, OTs, Speech and Language, and other agencies that contributed towards her final years. Elspeth was seriously ill for so long that I found it difficult to remember how things used to be before her illness. Now I have time to think, I begin to recall many great and happy memories from the early days. The one image that keeps coming back to my mind, though, is that of her following me around the bedroom with her eyes on our last day, as if she knew and was saying goodbye.

There was a lovely picture of a smiling Elspeth on the front cover of the funeral order of service, with her beautiful long red hair, which always stayed red and never went grey. That is how I will remember her, and the photo will now have a permanent position on the mantlepiece above the fireplace in my front room. I can see it clearly from where I sit, and it means that she will always be there. We wanted to grow old together, and we still can.

When we were first married, we used to go to the Suffolk coast for our holidays, and we would walk along beaches for hours, searching for amber, which had been washed up by the sea. We never found any. When I stood by Elspeth's coffin with the family at the end of the funeral service, I told her I would find her again. Perhaps one day we will walk on a beach together once more, and maybe we will, at last, find amber.

Milton Keynes UK
Ingram Content Group UK Ltd.
UKHW052026190824
447137UK00019B/298